ADULT
NURSING

Preparing for practice

Edited by

Dave Barton PhD MPhil BEd DipN RGN RNT

Head of Nursing , College of Human and Health Sciences, Swansea University, Swansea, Wales, UK and Chair, Association for Advanced Nurse Practitioner Education

Andrée le May BSc(Hons) RGN PhD PGCE(A)

Professor of Nursing, School of Health Sciences, University of Southampton

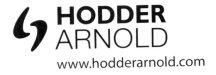
HODDER ARNOLD

www.hodderarnold.com

First published in Great Britain in 2012 by
Hodder Arnold, an imprint of Hodder Education, a division of Hachette UK
338 Euston Road, London NW1 3BH

http://www.hodderarnold.com

British Library Cataloguing in Publication Data
A catalogue record for this book is available from the British Library

Library of Congress Cataloging-in-Publication Data
A catalog record for this book is available from the Library of Congress

ISBN-13   978-1-444-11214-6

1 2 3 4 5 6 7 8 9 10

Commissioning Editor:	Naomi Wilkinson
Project Editor:	Joanna Silman
Production Controller:	Jonathan Williams
Index:	Lisa Footit

Cover images: Main image © Life in view/Science Photo Library. Top panel, left to right: Swansea University; Brian Bell/Science Photo Library; Pryzmat/iStockphoto; Deloche/Science Photo Library

Typeset in 11.25pt Adobe Garamond by Phoenix Photosetting, Chatham, Kent
Printed and bound in Italy

What do you think about this book? Or any other Hodder Arnold title?
Please visit our website: www.hodderarnold.com

ADULT
NURSING

To Miss Moos and Miss Jeffries -- Senior Nurse Tutors Kings College Hospital 1980 – who took a risk and accepted me to train as a Nurse. And to my student colleagues, the 'bright eyed and bushy tailed' gang of 50 who started that long career journey together.

DB

CONTENTS

SECTION TWO
Care themes and careers in nursing

CONTRIBUTORS

Maureen Coombs MBE, PhD, RN
Consultant Nurse Critical Care/Senior Lecturer in Nursing, Cardiac Intensive Care Unit,
Southampton General Hospital, Southampton

Heather Fillmore Elbourne RN, PhD
Dalhousie University, Geriatric Medicine, Halifax, Nova Scotia, Canada

Mary Gobbi RGN, Dip NEd, Dip N RNT, MA, PhD
Senior Lecturer, Faculty of Health Sciences, University of Southampton, Southampton

Steve Jones RMD, DipN (Land), Cert Ed FE (Wales), BA(Open), MBA (EBMs
Swansea)
Nurse Lecturer, Department of Nursing, School of Health Science, Swansea University,
Swansea

Elaine Lennan RGN, BN, MSc, PhD
Consultant Nurse, Southampton University Hospitals Trust, University of Southampton,
Southampton

Mike McIvor BSc (Hons), MSc (Nursing), RMN, RGN, RNT, PGCE (FE), Cert
in A&E Nursing
Lecturer, Department of Interprofessional Health Care Studies, School of Human and Health
Sciences, Swansea University, Swansea

Judith Morgan RGN, MA, CPE, BSC, ONC, CMS
Consultant Nurse in Emergency Care, Local Accident Centre, Neath Port Talbot Hospital, Port
Talbot

Carmel Sheppard RGN, BSc (Hons) Nursing Studies, MSc Professional
and Policy Studies, DBMS
Consultant Nurse/Lead Clinician Breast Cancer, Portsmouth Hospitals NHS Trust/University of
Southampton, Southampton

Jane Thomas SRN, RM, RHV, DipN (Wales), RNT/PGCE, MSc PH HP
Deputy Head of College of Human and Health Sciences, Swansea University, Swansea; and
Superintendent of Assessment, UKPHR Reviewer

Pauline Turner BA (Hons), RGN, MPhil, Diploma in Palliative Nursing
Retired Lecturer in Nursing, Faculty of Health Sciences, University of Southampton,
Southampton

FOREWORD

When my family heard that I planned on becoming a nurse their reaction was, "great, the world will be your oyster!" By this they meant that the qualification would give me the ability and freedom to do a wide variety of roles or go anywhere in the world. Their prediction was right as I have had a very varied career covering clinical practice, education and research. I have worked at national policy level and in other countries. Their comment is as true today for someone entering the nursing profession as it was all those years ago when they said it to me. If you are taking the first steps of your nursing career, I hope you feel excited about the many directions your practice could take. However, having a wide range of possibilities means you are faced with making choices, which can be hard, and this is where a book such as this comes in.

It is both exciting and daunting when considering what job to take or career path to follow. Many newly qualified nurses look for roles in areas they enjoyed during their initial education programme and may be reluctant to seek a role in areas they were not exposed to. This is in fact what I chose to do when I qualified; I sought the 'known' rather than the 'unknown' to begin my career. This is a perfectly sensible thing to do, as I knew I would be happy in my first professional role, however perhaps if I had been able to access information about what it is like to nurse in different specialities I may have made other choices. The chapters in this book will give you insights into the realities of practice in key areas of adult nursing and help you make informed decisions.

Looking back over my career and reflecting on the many conversations I have had with nurses about career options, I offer the following as some observations:

- The fear of the unknown is likely to influence the choices you make so think about gaining more information before dismissing an option out of hand.
- It is important to be honest with yourself about your personal likes and dislikes to ensure you get a good personal fit with a role. Generally speaking unhappy nurses make poorer carers.
- If possible try to access real life personal accounts of what it is like to work in a speciality – the case studies in this book are an excellent source.
- Career ladders and frameworks give a slightly misleading picture – many people move between roles and specialities that are at the same pay grade as well as moving upwards in pay grade. It may well be that through your life your career will change tack not once but many times as your aspirations and commitments change.
- Once established as a registered nurse, consider 'shadowing' someone who is doing a role you like the sound of. This will mean negotiating time away

from your workplace but is worth the effort as you can both observe the role first-hand and ask questions of the practitioner doing the job.

- Undertaking short secondments to experience a role for a limited period of time is also worth considering. This enables you to try out new roles without necessarily giving up your substantive post.

This book also underlines the importance of lifelong learning. Initial education programmes give you the grounding but developing expertise in your nursing practice is a career-long activity. Keeping up-to-date in order to function as a competent registrant is a requirement of your registration with the Nursing and Midwifery Council. Investing time in any training or education programme needs to be done with some careful thought, particularly around how it will improve your practice and how it will support your long term career aspirations.

Nursing is a wonderful profession as it not only enables us to make real and important differences to the lives of the people in our care but it opens up a world of opportunity. I finish with a quote by Albert Einstein:

Anyone who has never made a mistake has never tried anything new.

We should not be afraid to try new things; it is through experience that we grow as individuals.

Jean White
Chief Nursing Officer
Department Health, Social Services and Children, Welsh Government

October 2011

ACKNOWLEDGEMENTS

Dave Barton would like to thank the following nursing students from the Department of Nursing, College of Human and Health Sciences, Swansea University, who contributed some of their experiences for chapter 2: Monique Beavis (1st year student nurse), Sara Davies (2nd year student nurse), Sophie Evans (3rd year student nurse) and Julie Davies (newly registered staff nurse).

USING THIS BOOK AND COMPANION WEBSITE

The chapters in *Adult Nursing: preparing for practice* have been written to bring together an understanding of the principles of care in each area, the evidence base for practice (from research, policy, theory and experience) and information about the career pathways open to nurses. You will see the following features throughout the book:

OVERVIEW

Each chapter starts with an overview that explains the key topics in that area and what will be covered in the chapter.

About the authors

The editors have selected authors with significant expertise in their area of practice. These author biographies explain their career pathways to help you think about your development and future in nursing.

PROFESSIONAL GUIDELINES

Professional Guidelines are taken from key professional documents such as NHS policies, the Nursing and Midwifery Council code and so on.

STORY BOX

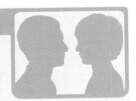

The experiences of student and practising nurses, patients and their relatives and carers are used throughout to bring theory to life. These 'voices' and case histories will help you relate what you learn to your own practice .

KEY POINTS AND EXPLANATIONS ARE HIGHLIGHTED IN GREEN BOXES.

ACTIVITY

To help you explore the topics and develop your practice, activities are included throughout. These include questions that encourage reflective thinking, signpost you to other sources of information or ask you to respond to a case history.

Accessing the resources on the companion website

Resources supporting this book are available online at www.hodderplus.co.uk/adult nursing.

These include:

- Interactive multiple choice questions (MCQs). Each test is scored so you can identify the areas to go back and revise.
- PowerPoint presentations which summarise the practical elements of each chapter for revision and learning. Separate presentations provide summaries of career development pathways.
- Ask the author: submit questions and the answers will be posted online.

To access these materials, go to www.hodderplus.co.uk/adult nursing and click on 'additional resources' in the right hand menu.

The first time you visit the website, you will need to register with your serial number. There is a link for this below the log in box.

Serial number: 904h3kwoht97

Once you have registered you will not need the serial number but can log in using your email address and the password you set up during registration.

Chapter 1

INTRODUCTION AND HOW TO USE THIS BOOK

Dave Barton, Andrée le May

This textbook is unique in its approach to furthering learning as it provides an evidence-based approach to care and showcases the breadth and intricacy of nursing careers. *Adult Nursing: Preparing for Practice* is designed to inspire final-year nursing students and new graduates to not only provide the best possible evidence-based care, but also to be excited by the many career opportunities in practice, management, education and research that nursing has to offer, all of which develop the best possible care for people.

This book is about taking your knowledge of nursing beyond the fundamentals that you will have covered in your initial years of education. There are sister texts to this one designed to help beginning students to get to grips with these fundamentals of practice – the skills, attitudes and knowledge that are critical to gaining registration and delivering high-quality care (Baillie, 2009; Hinchliff et al., 2008). This book is designed to help final-year students and newly qualified nurses to 'step up' to the role of a qualified nurse and subsequently structure their careers. Knowing how best to do this is particularly important in light of the recent national initiatives for the development of clinical and research career pathways and the extensive range of options that are now available to you as a qualified nurse.

Making the decision to have a career as an adult nurse is, in itself, an exciting move – once you near graduation you will be wondering what to do next – and many of you will keep wondering that throughout your careers! This book is about helping you to see the breadth of opportunity that is available to you throughout a career in nursing, be that in practice, management, education and/or research. In addition, we hope to help you to develop your expertise within a number of specialties in order to become an expert practitioner and develop the best possible care for those you encounter in your working life.

The book is divided into two sections. The first section – 'The world of nursing in modern-day healthcare' – is designed to:

- draw out key aspects of the journey from student to consultant practitioner, researcher, manager or teacher;
- present an overview of current career pathways and key roles in modern nursing. We use short case studies from people working in some of these roles throughout the book to bring the text to life;

- emphasise the key principles underpinning contemporary nursing in the UK. Here, we will draw on the four dimensions of practice essential, in our eyes, for sound professional practice regardless of career direction (skilled professional practice, leadership, research utilisation, and personal development and the development of others).

However, we believe that this section on its own is insufficient to show you how various careers impact on the delivery of high-quality care – only by showcasing career paths and linking them to particular aspects of care can we really demonstrate to you how exciting nursing can be and how the best possible care can be provided. In order to do this, we have designed a second section, written by practitioners, managers, researchers and educators, that melds aspects of their own career development, patient stories and the best available evidence from research, experience, policy and theory for practice.

This second section – 'Care themes and careers in nursing' – comprises six chapters loosely based around what have become known as the 'Darzi themes': first contact, access and urgent care; supporting long-term and palliative care; acute and critical hospital care; mental health and psychosocial care; and public health and primary care. These themes, although originating in the UK, have relevance across the world.

The authors in this section range from consultant nurses, through lecturers to postgraduate students. What unifies them is their level of expertise and their excitement about their work as nurses. The chapters do not cover everything that you need to know about each of the themes: rather, each of the authors has chosen to present to you the key aspects of care that they consider to be of most importance, particularly to newly qualified nurses. (If you want to delve into other areas of that particular specialty that interests you, key texts for further reading are given throughout.)

These key aspects range from learning how a sea-change in accepted principles of treatment and care led mental health nursing on a course divergent from acute hospital nursing, and that professional expectations nurtured in the physical care environment are likely to be challenged when caring for people with mental illness (see Chapter 9). In Chapter 5, you can learn more extensively about the intricacies of unscheduled care and how variety and autonomy are at the heart of working in this specialty. The need to become an advocate for older people admitted to acute care settings as well as a skilled expert nurse focusing on creating care, and environments, that nurture person-centredness shines through in Chapter 6, while the breadth of public health nursing and its impact on people and populations is palpable in Chapter 10. Chapter 7 captures the essence of nursing people with long-term conditions, and Chapter 8 shows how to face critical decisions and challenges as part of everyday nursing in critical care.

All of these chapters show how flexibility and courage lie at the heart of nursing decision-making and complement the application of a strong evidence base to practice. In each chapter, you can see how opportunities for professional development may occur in an unexpected form, in unlikely places and at a time when you may not feel prepared to take them on – this is particularly apparent in Chapter 9. Every chapter in this book places the nurse and the patient/client/service-user at its core.

We anticipate your using this book in a number of ways. Some of you will just want to dip into it to see what goes on in a particular specialty; others will want to look at the career stories embedded in each of the chapters and think about how these relate to your own careers or your aspirations; and there will be still others of you who want to use this book explicitly as a means to furthering your own practice development, to grow your expertise in certain aspects of nursing. We have tried to encourage readers to interact with the materials presented – we have exercises for you to do, multiple choice questions to answer and a web-based site that gives you more information and summary PowerPoint presentations of the chapters. But most of all we want you to be inspired to develop your nursing expertise, to develop your careers and, by doing both of these things, to develop the profession of nursing itself.

Read on …

References

Baillie L (ed.) (2009) *Developing Practical Adult Nursing Skills*. London: Hodder Arnold.

Hinchliff S, Norman S, Schober J (eds) (2008) *Nursing Practice and Health Care: A foundation text*. London: Hodder Arnold.

SECTION ONE
The world of nursing in modern-day healthcare

Chapter 2

PLANNING YOUR NURSING CAREER – PATHWAYS, OPTIONS AND KEY ROLES IN MODERN NURSING

Dave Barton

LEARNING OUTCOMES

At the end of this chapter, you should be able to:

- **Visualise the important milestones in your early development as a nurse**
- **Identify the key influences and themes that will structure your future career development**
- **Identify nursing roles, attributes, specialties and levels of practice**
- **Be able to construct a provisional career map**

OVERVIEW

This chapter is divided into two distinct sections. Section One will take you on a brief tour of your experiences so far as a student nurse, making the assumption that you are now coming to the end of your studies in your third year, or are newly qualified. It will outline how that will shape your options for your future career as a qualified nurse. Remember that this book is primarily designed to show the diversity of nursing, and how your career options today are far wider than they were for previous generations of nurses.

Section Two explores a range of possible nursing roles and consequent nursing careers. I must, however, emphasise from the outset that this is not comprehensive – and indeed reading the section should explain why this cannot be so. As we have repeatedly said throughout Chapter 1, nursing is incredibly diverse, and the depth of the scope of nursing roles and career pathways in the modern nursing profession is complex. Thus, this section at best touches on roles and pathways that are more commonly known and understood. However, there are many highly specific and singular nursing roles, and these will not be alluded to. So I apologise in advance if you find that not every possible role or career is detailed. However, you will find in the second section of the book more detailed descriptions of specialist areas of practice and specific roles.

About the author

I started my career as a student nurse at Normanby College of Nursing and Midwifery, Kings College Hospital, in 1980. On qualifying I took a staff nurse post on a neuromedical ward that specialised in multiple sclerosis and unstable epilepsy. I then moved to Intensive Care at Kings, dealing with general trauma and cardiothoracic surgery, where I also undertook specialist training in this area of practice. After moving to Wales in 1985 I worked in intensive care units in Carmarthen and in Swansea, and gained further experience in neurology and burns intensive care.

In 1990 I completed a Diploma in Nursing, and took a post as a Junior Tutor at the West Glamorgan School of Nursing and Midwifery. By 1992 I had completed a Degree in Education, and further developed my educational skills, involved in both pre-registration and post-registration studies. Throughout this I maintained my clinical skills by returning to practice on a regular basis. I completed an MPhil in 1995 and started to develop a keen interest in the development of nurse practitioners. Working closely with the RCN, I developed a national reputation as an educational expert in areas of advanced practice, and in the 2000s was the Chair of the National Association of Advanced Nursing Practice Educators, this representing the interests of over 40 UK Universities. In 2005 I gained my doctorate, and in 2007 became the Head of the Department of Nursing at Swansea University. I continue to publish widely and continue to return to clinical practice as often as I can.

Section One: Where do you start? Start at the beginning! So you wanted to be a nurse

You will by now have realised that nursing is a 'big' profession, and this 'bigness' manifests itself in many different ways. In terms of the sheer number of nurses, it is by anyone's estimation big. In the UK, there are 600 000 qualified nurses (Nursing and Midwifery Council, 2008a). The scale of that figure – over half a million nurses – says, if nothing else, that modern society clearly has a need for nurses. But what do they all do? The nursing profession must be one of the most diverse in the world, ranging from high-technology care in intensive care to community care, from caring for the very young to the very old, from working with people of great affluence to those in extreme poverty, from birth to death, encompassing every culture and belief. It seems that nursing offers a bewildering scope of career opportunities: clinical, management and leadership, education and research. But one thing is absolutely certain, it always starts from the same place – the day came you decided 'I want to be a nurse'.

I have for many years had the good fortune to interview potential candidates for nursing courses. Without exception, I always ask the one simple question that sets the scene for the rest of the interview – 'So – why do you want to be a nurse?' I have received so many different answers that I could not possibly reproduce them all here. Nevertheless, there is a pervading theme that can be identified in the successful applicant, that being the candidate's expressed desire to want to look after people. It is intriguing that so many candidates say this in an almost apologetic tone, whereas for me (as an experienced interviewer and a nurse) it is probably one of the most important traits that I am looking for in anyone who wants to become a nurse. Without finding that fundamental principle of wanting to care, I would have great misgivings about offering a candidate a place. If I had to pick out the best answer I ever had, this was from an enthusiastic young woman who was already a care assistant:

> Me: 'OK, so why do you want to be a nurse?'
> Candidate: 'Because I just love looking after people, and I think it is such a privilege to be allowed to wash someone.'

Needless to say I offered her a place.

However, having made the simple decision of wanting to embark on a nursing career, what follows will prove to be a little more complicated. It is not this book's intention to delve into the nuances of applying to be a nurse; I am assuming that you are already on your way through your studentship. (If this is not the case, we have provided some information for potential applicants to nursing in our online web resource.) Nor is it the intention to provide a comprehensive accompaniment to the curricula used in nursing undergraduate courses. There are plenty of texts on the shelves, some weighty tomes, that will take you through every aspect, theoretical and clinical, of your education while a student nurse. Rather, it is our intention to map out for you the modern career pathways of the nursing profession. To that end, and for the sake of completeness, I shall begin at the beginning: those of you who are already senior students or newly qualified nurses will have a chance to reflect on your early thoughts about learning nursing and your own experiences.

Fields of practice

You will already have decided from the outset whether you want to be an Adult, Child, Mental Health or Learning Disability Nurse (Box 2.1). These 'fields of

---

BOX 2.1   REGISTRANT FIELDS OF NURSING PRACTICE

THE ADULT NURSING FIELD

Adult Nurses, by definition, work with adults. However, they work in all areas of care, from community to hospital, with adults of all ages, and with diverse health problems and conditions ranging from the most acute to those involving long-term chronic illnesses.

Adult nursing is immensely diverse and demands skills of caring, communication, management, sensitivity, counselling, teaching and above all compassion and professionalism.

The Adult Nurse's knowledge of human illness is far-reaching, dealing with a vast array of physical conditions with an equally vast range of illness responses.

THE CHILDREN'S NURSING FIELD

Children's Nurses focus on the uniqueness of children and acknowledge that they are not simply 'little adults'. Children have particular developmental needs, and nursing this group will include building relationships and involving their families when the children receive nursing care.

Children's unique needs are defined by physical development, development of communication, emotional development, educational development and the need for a safe environment. The Children's Nurse is responsive and knowledgeable on those issues and provides care in partnership with the child's family in all social and care settings.

It is important to note that a child's response to physical illness may markedly differ from that of an adult.

THE LEARNING DISABILITY NURSING FIELD

Learning Disability Nurses care for people who have a wide range of physical and mental health conditions. They provide specialist support for families, carers and patients, and build partnerships that maximise independence. Social inclusion and well-being are the crucial foundations of practice, and the Learning Disability Nurse seeks to enable independence and equality of opportunity by overcoming physical and social barriers.

Learning Disability Nurses practise in a wide variety of settings, in residential and community centres, in patients' homes, in the workplace, and in schools and within adult education. They work with patients of all ages.

THE MENTAL HEALTH NURSING FIELD

Mental Health Nurses deal with a complex and demanding area of care. One in three people will experience a mental health problem in their life, and the range of conditions is extensive, including neuroses, psychoses and psychological and personality disorders.

Mental illness may occur as a result of a physiological change or life-changing event, or in reaction to some long-term social problem such as alcohol or substance abuse. The function of the Mental Health Nurse is to support patients and families, forming therapeutic relationships and enabling recovery where possible. They work mostly in community and social settings, although there are some areas of specialist and acute hospital service.

practice' (previously known as branches) structure your general and specific learning outcomes on the pre-registration programme. After 3 years of intense theoretical and clinical study, they will define your eventual formal registration as a nurse with the national regulator, the Nursing and Midwifery Council (NMC).

Interestingly, many countries around the world do not have specified fields of practice at pre-registration level, but educate all pre-registration nurses to a generic level of practice first. Subsequently, following formal qualification and registration, nurses then move into areas of specialisation. But here in the UK, it was decided back in the 1980s that we would have four fields (branches) of practice at pre-registration level, with the opportunity for further diverse specialisation once formally qualified.

This early 'pre-registration' specialisation will have required you, as a prospective candidate, to have done some homework very early on, before application and interview. You will have had to select which field of practice you aimed to apply for in advance, and thus have had some understanding of the differences between them. Adult nursing represents 80 per cent of the nursing workforce, with mental health, child and learning disability absorbing the remaining 20 per cent. You will have needed to know how these fields differed, and to have been clear at interview why you selected the field you wish to take.

In addition, pre-registration nursing degree programmes are most often designed to run over a 3-year period of full-time study. There are however many variations, such as family-friendly part-time options, cadet options, or shortened programmes where Assessment of Prior Learning may apply. Admission staff are well versed in this, and university websites are full of information on the individual nature of all these programmes. Making sure you were adequately prepared for your interviews was, I am sure, a priority. On the companion website for this book (see p. xiii for access details), we list some important points about interviews in general.

Being a student

You will by now be familiar with the structure and delivery of the programme you are attending. But do remember that pre-registration nursing degrees are structured, delivered and assessed in a variety of ways. Indeed, nursing programmes are undergoing considerable change at the time of writing (2011), moving away from Common Diploma Foundation and Specialist Branch structures to more integrated singular degree programmes defined by the use of generic and field competencies.

All pre-registration nursing programmes are assessed and validated by the national regulator, the NMC, and prospective nurses must meet the NMC competency outcomes before registration. The programme 'validation' process requires the university to demonstrate that its courses are fit for practice, meeting rigorous conditions for competencies, content, teaching and student support both in the clinical setting and

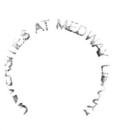

in the classroom. Without that validation, the university cannot run a programme. In addition, every programme must meet the demands of what are known as 'European Directives' for nursing. These directives specify common content and standards for all pre-registration nursing education programmes throughout the European Community, and thus enable qualified nurses to move around freely in these countries.

Validation by a central national regulator inevitably brings some conformity to the nature of pre-registration nursing programmes across the UK. Nevertheless, programme designs will vary from one university to the next as each institution puts together the degree structure in its own particular way, and in accordance with its own academic regulations. In almost all cases, programmes will follow the modular mode of delivery (where 'modules' are discrete units of learning that are individually assessed). However, every university will design its modules in different ways. For example, although the NMC stipulates that all students must spend 50 per cent of their time in clinical practice and 50 per cent of their time studying, universities will structure clinical practice and theory into their programmes and modules in different ways in conjunction with their clinical placement providers.

Your studentship is a hectic journey, but this is just the beginning of a long career that could take you many places. After 3 years of study and practice, and having successfully completed all the demands of your degree, you will begin your career as a qualified nurse, and in Section Two we will consider some of the options open to you in terms of future career pathways. What is certain is that you will have experiences that many people never encounter in a lifetime. Nursing is a demanding profession, and the way forward is always challenging. Even after 30 years of being a nurse, I am constantly surprised by new situations and unexpected learning curves.

THE STUDENT NURSE'S JOURNEY

Year 1

You will always remember your early days as a new student. A sea of new faces, new students, new friends, new lecturers, lots of uncertainties, lots to learn, and a bewildering array of sessions on student life, regulations, academic standards and clinical placements.

In your first year, you rapidly evolved from a complete novice to a junior student nurse. It is important to remember that this happened despite your having any previous relevant life or work experiences. Many student nurses have previously worked in care settings and held down responsible jobs; they may also be mature and have a family. All of this contributes to each person's learning and experience. But we all start from the same place, as a novice student nurse. People are not just born nurses; we have all had to undertake a great deal of learning and practice in order to acquire the skills and competencies that enable us to work successfully as qualified Registered Nurses.

In this first year of study, there were many fundamental skills that you needed to acquire. These included learning to move patients safely, basic management of violent or aggressive patients, feeding patients, taking blood pressure and other vital signs, learning to dispense medicines, and ensuring that all measures are taken to prevent cross-infection. As the dignity and humanity of our patients is paramount, you learned how this could be achieved in the busy and very real world of clinical practice. Theory underpins practice, and today's nurses explore the nature of our society, social order, psychology, sociology – these provide a foundation for understanding the complexity of the individual and society. Anatomy and physiology, pathology and the application of pathology underpin our understanding of the function of the human body. And the skills of critical thinking and analysis enable us to explore and examine the evidence that supports and directs nursing care.

Clinical practice provided hands-on care, in either acute or community settings, such as in a nursing home, in a general practice environment with practice nurses, district nurses and nurse practitioners, or in an acute medical or surgical ward with experienced hospital staff and specialist nurses. Clinical mentorship with experienced qualified nurses enabled you to gain the competencies required at that stage of your education.

Your early development should have been characterised by growing confidence. The first months were marked by 'firsts' – your first bed bath, your first injection, your first dressing, and your first grateful patient. There were the patients who were the first to tell you how wonderful you were, and those who were anything but complimentary. There was the first late shift, the first weekend shifts, the first ward reports, the first assignments, and perhaps even the first experience of death. Nursing is so diverse and complex that even though certain skills become increasingly second nature and routine, there is always something just around the corner that will be another 'first'. I can vouch for this – after all my time as a nurse, I am still having 'firsts'!

In your first year, you took the first steps to becoming a qualified nurse and may have discovered areas of practice that you favoured over others. It is important to hold on to those first impressions, nurture them and see how they relate to later experiences in nursing. These may be influential in guiding your future career choices.

I commenced my nursing training as a mature student after completing a higher education course in health studies. This course worked in conjunction with the local university's nursing degree and gave me an idea of what standard of work was expected.

As a mature student juggling university and a home life (particularly as a mother of four), time management was vitally important to me. Fortunately, I was used to managing my time well as, prior to the commencement of my course, I had worked as a complementary therapist, so I was used to organising my family's childcare.

I believe being a mature student has benefited me as I have a different outlook on life; my enthusiasm for the course shows through in my attitude towards all aspects of the course, and gives me the ability to relate to all ages within the university and on practical placements.

During the first month of my first year as a student nurse, I underwent a major transition and realised that undertaking this course would be the most challenging process I would ever experience. Despite this, my commitment and dedication to the course was paramount. I felt overwhelmed by the amount of information and learning it entailed. The lectures and the amount of time I had to spend at university were relatively intense, but as my first month ran into my second I began to settle into the structure of the course, gaining confidence and enjoying learning and practising the skills and competencies that I would need to enable me to commence my first placement. I enjoyed all features of the course and have benefited from attending lectures and the learning events preceding placements. Attending each lecture and practical session has given me the groundwork for nursing as a first-year student, taking me to a higher level of academic learning in each practical placement.

At each placement, I see a new page of 'my nursing life' waiting to be written on and to be carried forward onto the next page. I am always eager to learn and expand my knowledge, listening to senior staff and benefiting from their many years of experience. Although during my first placements I found I was working only on instruction from senior members of staff, I soon started to form my own opinions on the situations that arose.

I have gained a wide range of knowledge from my diverse practical placements. Practice placements are tiring, but you gain invaluable hands-on experience and get back what you put in. I have worked in various clinical areas including the outpatient department, a nursing home, and a community placement where I worked alongside a health visitor, district nurses and a practice nurse – this allowed me the opportunity to care for a wide age range of people from all walks of life who were experiencing varying health issues.

The time I spent with the district nurses gave me insight into a service that provides specialist advice and support for patients and their families in their homes. This helps them to be aware of community services and of their own anticipated needs, and enables them to make informed decisions about realistic care and autonomy in decision-making. Throughout this experience, I realised the importance of good communication between hospital and community staff, which taught me that methods of communication and interaction between professions and patients are imperative. Since my first placement, I have greatly improved my own communication skills, and my confidence has grown.

During my first year as a student nurse, the support and advice I got from tutors and mentors was welcome: whether it was related to the course or to any other aspect of life, it ensured that I and my peers progressed with our studies. This assurance and support has helped me develop into a confident and responsible student nurse, which I believe has been reflected in my practical placements, making me always aware of the safety and welfare of patients. Successful communication with tutor and mentors is vitally important as they offer assistance with assignments and documentation; I feel that I can self-assuredly approach them with any issue, whether academic or personal, but I always envisage their time limitations. All students need to be able to rely on their superiors at some point during the course, and mine have always been there, showing encouragement and criticism when appropriate, which has facilitated me in the success I have achieved throughout my first year.

Although I have a excellent network of support from my superiors, much of the support comes from my peers. As a mature student, I felt, at first, a little out of my comfort zone as many of the students are fresh out of school and college, and being so much older than the majority of them, I felt a little intimidated. However, this feeling was eradicated with the realisation that everyone had the same agenda as me – to flourish into the best nurse they could possibly be.

From a young age, I always wanted to become a nurse, but as life takes the path it takes, situations arise that are out of your control, and the idealistic takes a back seat. I have worked since leaving school over 16 years ago, but I have always thought about the 'what ifs'. Taking the decision to return to college was a very daunting experience, and taking that step was the biggest one I have ever taken. Although I wish I had pursued this dream many years ago, I am in other ways glad I waited as my dedication towards nursing is greater now than ever, and I can give more to the career I have chosen.

As I am about to start my second year, the experiences I have been through in my first year have confirmed absolutely my choice to pursue a nursing degree. Starting the second year is going to be exciting, and I hope the enthusiasm and commitment I bring with me excel. I believe that nursing is my vocation and not simply my occupation.

YEAR 2

In year 2, you began to climb what is a long ladder (nursing has a big hierarchy!), and first-year students looked on you as a senior – even though you may not have felt that you were. The pressure of assessment was relentless, and you were now realising that the more you knew, the more you realised you didn't know. In reality, you were beginning to refine and utilise your developing skills more widely, although you may not have known it.

Your skill of communicating with patients with a spectrum of difficulties and disorders was increasing, and you will have developed a broader view of working in a multiprofessional environment, working and communicating with doctors, physiotherapists, pharmacists and all the other many professionals that can comprise a team. You may unfortunately have seen examples of poor practice as well as good practice. It is crucial that you remember that there is much to be learnt by seeing things done badly and other critical incidents. Although we (obviously) do not in any way condone poor practice, and we strive to provide only the very best of care, we realistically acknowledge that poor practice can happen, and that students may see this. I have seen students return to their personal tutorial groups and reflect at some considerable length, and in depth, on the issues that have troubled them. It is to be hoped that this has enabled them to understand and learn from these experiences in such a way that it has improved their practice and ultimately improved the profession itself.

However, it would not do for me to place too much emphasis on learning from negative experiences. More positively, you will have seen how well nursing can improve quality of life. In my experience, good nursing predominates in practice, and in my travels through clinical areas, I am constantly confronted by the highest quality of nursing practice – and that is as it should be.

A SECOND-YEAR STUDENT'S STORY – SARA DAVIES

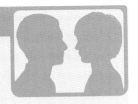

I commenced my nursing training immediately upon completion of my 'A' level course at a comprehensive school. During this time, I benefited from having work experience at a residential home for the elderly.

The structure of my second year is almost identical to that of my first year. A slight difference, however, is the increase in duration of placements and lectures by 1 week each, and the increased depth of evaluation and learning. I enjoy both aspects and benefit from attending lectures prior to each placement. The learning process gives me confidence and allows me to question my own actions and judgements in order to improve my practice. This year, I feel capable of offering opinions rather than acting solely on instructions, as was the case in my first year, when I learned as much as possible but did not formulate my own opinions, although I did take a personal note of situations where I would have operated differently. My increased experience and confidence allow me to voice my difference of opinion and, in so doing, hopefully benefit patients.

I am now more accountable for my actions and have developed from being a junior student accepting instructions without question into a senior student who has the confidence and experience to skilfully question practices that appear to require change. However, it is vitally important to be aware of my own level of knowledge and competency and not go beyond these limits.

My second year gives me a wide range of knowledge through experience in different placements. I have worked on various hospital wards, observed a range of operations in theatre and spent time with district nurses and health visitors. This has all allowed me opportunities to care for people within a wide age range suffering from varying health problems. As a student in a Welsh university, I have benefited from being bilingual and have learnt that communication with a patient in his or her mother tongue can be beneficial, resulting in improved understanding, increased patient confidence and the development of a more responsive rapport.

Despite maturing in knowledge and experience during my second year, I continue to welcome the support and advice available from my mentors and tutor. Throughout this period, I have benefited from their assurance that I am making positive developments in my awareness of my responsibility for the safety and well-being of patients. I can confidently approach my mentors for advice and support but am always aware of time constraints and the need to make prior arrangements for any discussions. Sound organisation and a respect for my superiors ensure that a successful working relationship develops with my mentors and tutor. Both provide backing for the paperwork involved in assignments and documentation, and this support improves my academic skills and gives me confidence to persevere independently and achieve the best standards of presentation. Students rely upon the crucial support of mentors and tutors to achieve success, and I am grateful to mine for their encouragement and for the caring relationship, which is growing and maturing during my second year.

Working within a multidisciplinary team offers a variety of responsibilities and the need to adapt to a range of tasks in different clinical circumstances. These demands are challenging but provide opportunities that supersede these challenges and create a feeling of great satisfaction. Some examples of this include the ability to care for people of different backgrounds, to deal with a range of medical problems and to adapt to a mixture of placements.

My character and personality have benefited from association with students of varying ages and from different backgrounds. Progressing from comprehensive school to university did not present any difficulties and, to my satisfaction, I have made many friends within my circle of students that I would have deemed improbable 2 years ago. During placements, I also meet third-year students. Their enthusiasm and dedication have given me encouragement and an incentive to progress to my third year.

From an early age, I favoured a nursing career. My first year at university positively confirmed my choice, but my second year has given me the inspiration and stimulus to confidently pursue a nursing career, as well as the satisfaction of choosing a vocation worthy of my best endeavour. One highlight of my second year is being chosen to join 14 students on a month's visit to India within a Study Abroad Programme.

Year 3

By the end of the final year of your degree, nursing has become a part of your 'psyche', it's under your skin, you 'think' like a nurse, there starts to be an intuitive feel to your actions, and yet you are still beset by new experiences. Exposure to the more seriously and critically ill patients brings new perspectives. You take increasingly more responsibility for your own caseload, and that brings new authority – but with this will come new anxieties. You will have seen patients with a bewildering scope of health problems, in the home and in formal care, ranging from the minor to the truly catastrophic.

What is certain is that you are not the person that you were. And yet everything is now hanging precipitously as you move toward the programme's final conclusion. It is now that you will begin to identify areas of practice that you see yourself undertaking as a qualified nurse – and these thoughts are crucial for your future. Your university may well provide some formal sessions on career planning, or job fairs where prospective employers tout to fill vacancies in their organisations. What I would recommend is that you talk to your personal tutors and mentors both in the university and in clinical practice. Seek their advice and guidance, and weigh your options carefully. Although I accept that getting a job is the primary hurdle, try to look to the future and gauge where you will be (where you would want to be) in 5 or even 10 years. Some of the possible pathways available to you will be the subject of discussion throughout the later chapters of this book.

A THIRD-YEAR STUDENT'S STORY – SOPHIE EVANS

I am in the third and final year of my nursing degree, and I am amazed how the time has gone so quickly. It has certainly been a busy but enjoyable 3 years. While undertaking the degree, I have had a variety of clinical placements in both primary and acute settings. These placements have complemented the theoretical elements of the course and enabled me to develop the skills and knowledge required to become a staff nurse. I am currently on my critical placement in intensive care. I have found this placement very interesting, and I am beginning to understand the role of the nurse and the process of caring for patients who are critically ill and ventilated.

The nursing process has been a core component of my training, and therefore I now feel competent in assessing, planning, implementing and evaluating nursing care. I have now learnt always to include patients and their relatives where appropriate as it aids accuracy and facilitates the growth of a therapeutic relationship. Throughout my training, I have had increasing responsibilities for groups of patients, which has incorporated time management, prioritising care delivery, completing written documentation and giving verbal reports to colleagues. I have learnt when delivering patient care always to practise in a manner that maintains patient confidentiality and dignity, and I respect patient individuality and choice.

I understand the importance of policy adherence when administering medication and performing nursing procedures. So as I am to become a newly qualified staff nurse in a couple of months, I am now beginning to understand and know the scope of my capabilities – and of course I will always seek advice when I need to. I am a little nervous about the transformation of going from being a student to a qualified staff member – 'being in blue'! But I am looking forward to the challenge and gaining experience in 'the real world of nursing'.

Stepping into practice (and getting a job)

Getting your first post as a new staff nurse is a little daunting. Well, actually it's hugely daunting. The step from student nurse to qualified nurse cannot be understated. It is a momentous process of change, and this brings all the uncertainties and fears that processes of change bring. You will no longer have the safety net of 'being a student'. You will not have the option of turning to the lecturers and tutors when you are uncertain. You will be a qualified nurse, and your patients and the public will expect you to have the knowledge and expertise that would be expected of any nurse.

You have passed all your exams, all your assessments, all your competencies; you have experienced a rite of passage. But remember that a rite of passage is characterised by three very distinct phases. When you started as a student nurse in your first year, you had to start to separate from your previous identity and acknowledge that you were going to change and become a very different person. As you progressed through the programme, you experienced transition, moving from one state to another as you absorbed all the knowledge and experiences of your studentship. And now, as you step into practice, you have to incorporate a new identity as a fully fledged professional registered nurse. This is going to be stressful and will not happen instantly, but every nurse has experienced it, so don't be overly anxious. In a remarkably short period of time, you will find your feet, engage with your new professional identity and start your journey through the multicoloured and wonderful world of nursing.

However, a significant part of that final stage of your rite of passage is getting your first job as a qualified nurse. What is important is to be assertive, quietly, confidently assertive. It is really important to present yourself in the best possible way. A good CV is a good starting point, but your prospective employers will want to interview you, and just as you were well prepared for your university interview, be equally well prepared for your job interview(s). Do not limit yourself or put 'all your eggs into one basket'. Look around and apply for several posts. This does not put prospective employers off: it indicates that you are assertive and ambitious, professional qualities that are good to have.

I have had students say to me in the past, when asking about the content of a CV or prospective questions at an interview, 'But what do I say that I have done? I have been a student!' This is of course nonsense, as every part of your university course, both the theoretical and clinical components, have contributed to your development as a professional Registered Nurse. The fact that you have only just qualified is immaterial as you have much to offer. And getting that point across is crucial (see the box). Every interviewer will want to know why you have selected their hospital, their service, their specialty as the one that you want to start your career in. It's up to you to convince them that your reasons are good.

THE ELEMENTS OF THE JOB INTERVIEW FOR THE NEWLY QUALIFIED NURSE

Key interview preparation

Remember that the format of interviews can vary considerably. Some employers may use a simple face-to-face interview, while others may also include drug tests, patient scenarios and group discussions within the interview process. Make sure that you ask in advance what format the interview will take. This is important to know, and will allow you to start thinking about how you prepare for an interview.

- Don't ask for too much, you are going to be the most junior member of their team – balance ambition with contribution.
- Remember – you *are* a good team player.
- Expect the question 'Tell us about yourself'? This does not refer to your social life – they want to know about you as a professional nurse!
- Expect the question 'Why do you want to work here?'
- Expect the question 'What do you think are going to be the main challenges of being a newly qualified nurse?'
- Expect the question 'What are your strong points and weak points?' (Suggestion – a good weak point is that you are very concerned with getting care right. Weak points should always be presented in a positive light.)
- Expect the question 'Do you have anything to ask us?'
- Take in a list of questions. Even if your interviewers cover them all during the interview, refer to your list and tell them they have covered everything.

DAY 1: A QUALIFIED REGISTERED NURSE – SO WHAT HAPPENS NEXT?

You walk on to the ward, unit, clinic. You're a staff nurse – and this is your first day. It's a very strange feeling. The first thing you have to remember is 'DON'T PANIC'. Second, remember that, despite how you feel, you do not have a big sign hanging over your head saying 'FIRST DAY'. This you may or may not view as a good thing, but what is certain is that all the patients and public will see is a staff nurse.

A DIARY OF YOUR FIRST DAYS

Think back and remember those first few days as a new staff nurse.

Write the diary of those first days as if it were now. What were the key feelings that you had? What were your fears and hopes? What were your aspirations? What does that tell you about yourself now as a nurse?

There are many who believe that probationer periods are crucial for the newly qualified nurse (Nursing and Midwifery Council, 2008b), and indeed the NMC has indicated its desire to see this introduced as a mandatory requirement. Indeed, it is good employment practice that you are provided with a sensible induction programme that will ease you into your new role, support you in practice and ensure that all legal requirements in terms of in service training are met.

However, none of this will change your feelings of apprehension on day 1. And the real longer term question will be 'what next'?

EARLY DAYS AS A NEW STAFF NURSE – JULIE DAVIES

During my final 12 weeks of training to be a nurse, I was on a ward managing my own patients and workload under supervision from a qualified nurse acting as my mentor. At this stage, I was feeling confident with my actions and had knowledge and experience to relate theory to practical skills that I had to pass on to nursing students who were in early stages of their nursing programme as part of achieving final competencies.

I realised that I did not want to lose this new-found confidence and decided to start applying for jobs within my local NHS Trust. I began by compiling a curriculum vitae, as this would contain all relevant information and dates that a standard NHS application form would require. I was also warned on my nursing programme that I would be asked to produce a personal statement at the end of the application to promote my qualities, skills and experiences. As I gained experience of completing application forms, I discovered that reading the job description thoroughly was the key, and that adjusting each personal statement to suit the qualities and skills required for the job was an important aspect of fine-tuning my application.

Reality soon started to hit home that I was about to be a qualified nurse when I got offers of interviews. In order to prepare for these interviews, I read up on recent topics that were relevant to my local Trust, and on the criteria that were required and described within the job description. At interview, I found myself very nervous: trying to keep calm, collected and confident was difficult. Most questions asked of me were constructed using scenarios of events that could happen regularly on the ward. I always tried to take a minute before answering these questions as I had been involved in or witnessed most of the scenarios during my training. Therefore my answers involved me recalling events and always detailed how I would make sure that I was safe, that my patients were safe, and that if I did not know current policy, I would always seek advice from a senior colleague.

Receiving a job offer was very exciting. I remember feeling very proud, very privileged, but also being conscious that many of my fellow nursing students had not yet even experienced job interviews or applied for jobs. At the back of my mind, I always knew that the competition was going to be tough – which is why I started well ahead of some people. Nursing is a challenging and demanding profession, and it requires a lot of assertiveness and organisation skills to succeed. I soon realised that I had these skills and qualities as I prepared early and received a job offer before obtaining my degree classification and pin number.

Suddenly, the final day of my nursing programme was upon me. After 3 years of hard work, theory and endless essays, I had received my degree classification. All I was waiting for was my name to be forwarded by the university to the NMC. Within a week, I received that letter of welcome and a notification of registration fees. After receiving my degree classification, the whole process of registration took approximately 2 weeks. On payment of the NMC fee, I realised that 'this is it, I am registered and qualified to practise as a general nurse'; that's when I first discovered butterflies in my stomach.

My first day as a staff nurse was very scary. I was so nervous and worried as I thought that this would be it, me on my own. I felt stupid at times because all I appeared to do was ask questions. I would find myself being asked by doctors, patients and relatives questions that most of the time I could not answer. I thought I was never going to stop saying those four little words: 'I'll just find out.' However, my confidence began to grow, and I was assigned two mentors within 2 weeks of starting my employment, along with a new set of competencies to work through within my preceptorship. From a very early stage in my employment, I felt that I was receiving lots of support, advice and encouragement from my mentor and the ward sisters, for which I was very grateful.

Career options

Throughout this chapter, I have referred to there being many career options available to you as a nurse. Perhaps now is the time to actually state what they are, and begin some provisional discussion on what they mean. In this book, as is evidenced by the later chapters, we have made considerable use of the care pathways highlighted by Lord Darzi in his influential report (Department of Health, 2008) on the shape of the NHS and healthcare in the future (Box 2.2).

We have modified these care pathway themes slightly to meet the needs of our discussion on career options (career pathways), and it is not my intention now to deal with each of these. Section Two of this chapter will give you some further information on how careers may be mapped into roles, and each theme has an entire chapter devoted to it later in Section Two of the book.

BOX 2.2   CARE /CAREER PATHWAYS (MODIFIED FROM THE DARZI THEMES)

- Acute Care
- Unscheduled Care
- Chronic and Palliative Care
- Critical and Emergency Care
- Mental Health Care
- Public Health and Community Care
- Specialist and Advanced Practice (cuts across all of the above)

Darzi saw the focus on future patient care as defined by these areas of care, and indeed he envisaged the very structure of future healthcare as being built around them. For each of the areas of care, there would have to be resources provided, expertise developed and careers defined. Thus, in this book, we have taken the care themes and career pathways (the two being inextricably intertwined) as the basis for career development in nursing in the twenty-first century. Although these themes were fundamental to Darzi's vision of health reform, it is important to remember that they are not unique to healthcare in the UK: indeed, they are congruent with global health themes identified by others (e.g. the World Health Organization) and as such are likely to provide an enduring framework on which to structure discussions about health, not only in this book, but also in other media in the future.

The future of nursing careers has also been significantly influenced by the Modernising Nursing Careers initiative that published a report in 2010. The impact of this work is so important that I will now briefly review this, since much of what comes later in this book is built on its recommendations and presumptions.

MODERNISING NURSING CAREERS: SETTING THE DIRECTION

Each UK country has a Chief Nursing Officer (CNO) employed by the UK's government to give strategic advice on all matters that relate to nursing and its contribution to the health of the nation. In 2006, the four CNOs reviewed the status of nursing in the UK to determine its ability to respond to new and changing social and health needs, and found a need for considerable reform. As a result of that, they initiated the Modernising Nursing Careers project, and that complex work programme is still underway in 2011 and is setting the direction for the future of nursing over the next 30 years and beyond.

Modernising Nursing Careers crafted a vision for the future of the nursing profession in the twenty-first century. It wanted nurses to be able to provide and contribute to care in such a way that met the complexity of a modern and changing society that was being driven primarily by care delivery, as well as by politics, cost and technology. In future, the report suggested, nurses would need to respond to new health problems and needs, and progress in career pathways in such a way to make best use of their skills, ability and aspirations. The report identified a clear need for change to enable nurses to meet the demands arising from a modernised health service. Nurses, the report stated, should be able to 'work in different care settings, to take on changed roles and responsibilities, develop a varied mix of skills, to pursue education and training when they need it, and to develop both generalist and specialist skills as they require them' (Department of Health, 2006, p. 14).

The Modernising Nursing Careers report emphasised that the profession of nursing needed in the future to be seen as offering a modern, dynamic and fulfilling career. Nursing needed to acknowledge that prospective new recruits also had the choice of other professions, and that in such a competitive market it was crucial that the career framework reflected this. That framework had to meet the future care needs of patients by acknowledging the way in which the health services were changing and were likely to continue to do so.

I have outlined above how the Darzi themes in many ways define the career pathways that that you may select from. However, one of the important outcomes of Modernising Nursing Careers was the identification of new challenges for nurses in the future in response to the changing demands of society's health needs. All nurses will need to able respond to these challenges regardless of their specific career pathway. Later in this chapter, I will take this further and look in more detail at how these diverse demands translate into existing and new roles, as well as how career pathways may be 'mapped'.

PROFESSIONAL GUIDELINES

THE FUTURE DEMANDS FOR A MODERNISED NURSING WORKFORCE

In future the nursing workforce will need to:

- Organise care around the needs of patients
- Ensure patients have a good experience of nursing as reputations of organisations and patient choice will rest on the quality of nursing
- Work in a range of settings, crossing hospital and community care, and use telemedicine
- Have the skills and competencies to care for older people and people with long term conditions, who may have both physical and mental health needs
- Be able to use preventative and health promotion interventions
- Work for diverse employers, and take opportunities for self-employment where appropriate
- Have sufficient numbers of nurses with advanced level skills to meet demand
- Work as leaders and members of multidisciplinary teams inside and outside hospital, and across health and social care teams
- Work with new forms of practitioners, for example assistant practitioners and anaesthesia practitioners
- Deliver high productivity and best value for money.

(Department of Health, 2006, p. 10)

In addition to these proposals, Modernising Nursing Careers also identified other key challenges for the nursing profession if it were to meet the needs of a modern and changing health service and society. These focus on change, career advice, maintaining fitness to practice and recognising individual and organisational responsibilities.

CHANGE IS A FACT OF LIFE

The nursing profession must in future accept the need to change and evolve as it responds to the demand of the population it serves. It must respond to advances in treatments, advances in health technology and changes in service delivery, and respond to the need for new professional roles, as this quote from the *Post Registration Careers Framework in Wales* indicates.

> There is clear evidence that the population is ageing, with many older patients presenting with chronic/long term conditions and multiple health needs, while obesity is increasing in the younger members of society. The nursing workforce must therefore maintain a degree of flexibility, engaging fully with appropriate and ongoing development opportunities. (Welsh Assembly Government, 2008, p. 4)

CAREER ADVICE

The Modernising Nursing Careers report identified the need for a clear career framework within the profession, and that this framework needed to be understood by the public. This textbook is, in part, based on that recommendation.

FITNESS TO PRACTICE, BASED ON REGULAR APPRAISAL AND ONGOING PROFESSIONAL DEVELOPMENT

Modernising Nursing Careers reinforced the principle that had been established for some time in the Post-Registration Education and Practice (PREP) standard (Nursing and Midwifery Council, 2010). This standard has been coupled with the introduction of periodical re-registration to ensure that the Nursing Register reflects a 'live' list of practising nurses. It may today seem surprising to have to state that all Registered Nurses must continue to develop their skills and knowledge throughout their career, and to be able to provide evidence of that development, if they are to be allowed to continue to practice. However, it is a requirement that was only formally instituted within the nursing profession in the late 1980s. Prior to that date, there was no such requirement, and previously the Nursing Register included those who had long ceased to practise – or who had even long since passed away.

In the early 2000s we saw the introduction of the Agenda for Change agreement (Department of Health, 2004a) and the NHS Knowledge and Skills Framework (KSF; Department of Health, 2004b). These tools, used in conjunction with an appropriate peer reviewer, emphasise and structure the requirement for staff in the NHS to have professional development plans focusing on the following:

- the duties and responsibilities of the individual's post and current agreed objectives;
- the application of knowledge and skills in the workplace;
- the consequent development needs of the individual.

Attending to each of these is crucial for your future career development – and paying serious attention to them as part of your employment also means that your employer has a part to play in enabling your professional development plans.

But on that note, a reality check. I know some nurses who will respond with a hearty laugh to the notion of career development plans and annual reviews. In the reality of a busy hospital, clinic, ward or health centre, the niceties of such plans may go astray. However, it is also a reality that your future career as a nurse may depend on having such plans in place, and the NMC and employers are becoming increasingly focused on this as nursing roles evolve – particularly into areas of advanced practice. And with that point in mind, I move on to the responsibility of individuals in assuring their own fitness to practice.

INDIVIDUAL RESPONSIBILITIES

The profession of nursing is carefully regulated by Act of Parliament. Every Registered Nurse must comply with the requirements of the NMC Code of Conduct, Performance and Ethics (Nursing and Midwifery Council, 2008b). The Code demands and requires that Registered Nurses update and evaluate their knowledge, competence and skills throughout their careers.

In order to maintain registration, nurses must also comply with the NMC PREP standards (Nursing and Midwifery Council, 2008b). These standards clearly state that nurses must have worked for a minimum of 450 hours in a nursing capacity and undertaken 35 hours (5 days) of continuous professional development activity in the 3 years prior to renewal of their registration.

As a Registered Nurse, *you* are responsible for your personal development within your nursing career, wherever that career may take you.

ORGANISATIONAL RESPONSIBILITIES

However, it must also be acknowledged that organisations (employers) have a responsibility to ensure that their staff work in safe, appropriate environments. Part of that responsibility includes a demand that staff have the opportunity and support to develop expertise within their specific roles. The health services within the four countries of the UK all have policies that underpin this principle, and entrenched in these policies are the principles of planned and appropriate recruitment that enable staff to participate in induction and mandatory training programmes. There are also principles that enable staff to participate in ongoing professional development. Thus, there is a means by which professional development may be structured, and this is crucial for Registered Nurses who are responsible for meeting the PREP standards for periodical re-registration.

Section Two: Contemporary nursing careers – pathways and key roles in modern nursing

So how do you plan a nursing career, and what are the general options available to you? Previously in this chapter, we saw that, even for new students, nursing presents a vast and varied profession with what may seem to be a bewildering array of roles and areas of practice. Indeed, we have already seen that, in the pre-qualifying period, you will already have specialised into one of four fields of practice: learning disability, child, mental health or adult. Thus, it would seem that, at least in one sense, these four registrant fields define the career pathways for the future nurse. However, the boundaries between these fields are often blurred, and we see nurses caring for patients with multiple presentations: families with children, adults with physical and mental health problems, individuals with physical illness that results in disability. Thus, the initial registrant fields provide only part of the career structure; there are, in reality, far more factors to be considered.

It must also be acknowledged that many newly qualified nurses currently have little idea of where they see themselves in the future, above and beyond securing their first staff nurse post. Nevertheless, once you have that first post, the time will soon come when you say to yourself, 'What next?' Indeed, it is perhaps a failure of our current workforce planning that this is the case, when nurses should really have a clear view of their future and their contribution to healthcare. In short, we must move to a system where nursing careers are modernised, planned, professional and appropriate.

Recent national initiatives have looked closely at how nurses develop their practice once qualified, often moving to more advanced roles. This work has not been based just on what nursing wants as a professional career framework, but also on what the health service needs in the future from the nursing profession. For example, the NMC has constantly worked to refine and develop the guidance it gives to Registered Nurses, and has responded to the strategic changes and needs. The Darzi framework (Department of Health, 2008) has looked at the types or areas of care that currently predominate and those that will be significant in the future. In addition, the work of the Scottish Government, on behalf of the national Modernising Nursing Careers initiative, has considered the foundations and pillars that structure the development of nurses' roles as they advance through their careers (Department of Health, 2010). These strategic drivers have provided more clarity on the pathways and domains of practice open to new nurses.

Box 2.3 outlines these 'career domains'. First, there is the domain that represents the registrant fields (fields of practice), the parts of the Nursing Register that you are included in on qualifying and that legally allow you to practise as a nurse. These are controlled by Act of Parliament. Second, there is the domain that features predominating areas of care that are defining the health service – the areas of care that the public need demands. These have been highlighted by the Darzi Report, and I present them here in modified form. Finally, there is the domain that is structured on the foundational pillars of professional nurse role development as identified by the Modernising Nursing Careers agenda in its Advanced Practice Toolkit (Department of Health, 2010).

The question, however, relates to how you, the newly qualified nurse, will draw all these domains together to map and plan your career. Well, to start with, choose the areas that most apply to you, and those that most interest you; then make a map and see what it looks like. That map need not be set in tablets of stone. You may have several aspects that interest you, and they may become modified over time as your career develops and as opportunities arise. In Fig. 2.1, I give some examples of what these career maps may look like – doing these quick sketches will help you to see your interests more clearly and thereby plan your educational as well as employment journey in order to meet your career aspirations. As you can see, the maps can become more complex as your career develops, adding new components, or when one feature begins to dominate in a role.

This discussion would, however, be incomplete if we did not also consider salary. It is perfectly natural that, as individuals progress through their career and develop more complex skills and greater responsibilities, they expect a higher salary. Thus, for completeness, Box 2.4 outlines the current (at the time of writing, 2010–2011) Health Service pay bands – I will refer to this on occasion throughout the rest of this chapter in terms of where some nursing roles rank on the pay scales.

ACTIVITY

YOUR CAREER MAP

Plan out your career map as it is today. How does it compare with your ideas when you were a student or just newly qualified?

Career Map 1

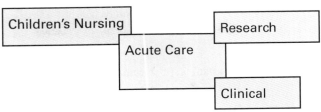

In this simple map, the nurse has selected Acute Care and Children's Nursing as the main areas of practice. The nurse has also noted a particular interest in Clinical work and Research.

Career Map 2

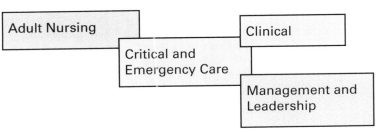

In this simple map, the nurse has selected Critical and Emergency Care and Adult Nursing as the main areas of practice. The nurse has also noted a particular interest in Management and Leadership in Clinical work.

Career Map 3

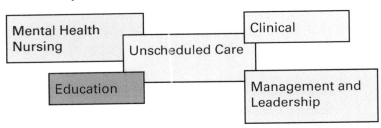

In this map, a more complex combination of Unscheduled Care and Mental Health has been selected as the main areas of practice. A particular interest in Education, and Management and Leadership in Clinical work are noted.

Career Map 4

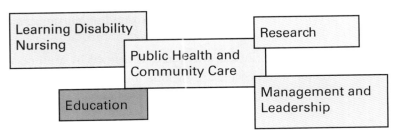

In this map, the nurse has again selected a more complex combination of Public Health and Community Care and Learning Disability Nursing as the main areas of practice. The nurse has also noted a particular interest in Education, and Management and Leadership in Clinical work.

Figure 2.1 An example of increasingly more complex career maps

Having set the scene, let us now move on to consider a number of key points and issues, and review some (but not all) established nursing roles. I will also review some topical but less well understood role developments in nursing. All these factors and roles are having an impact on the scope of practice of the nursing profession, and thus on the career direction of individual nurses. These factors are:

- nursing as a professional career;
- becoming a staff nurse – managing the transition;
- the clinical mentor (education and teaching in practice);
- the ward sister/charge nurse;
- the district nurse and the practice nurse;
- the advanced clinical nurse;
- the nurse prescriber;
- the nurse consultant;
- the nurse manager/nurse executive;
- the nurse educator;
- the nurse researcher.

NURSING AS A PROFESSIONAL CAREER

In every text you have read on nursing, in every book and journal, you will have seen nursing referred to as a profession. But have you ever asked yourself what constitutes a 'profession'? Plumbers are often referred to as professionals, as are electricians, builders and decorators. We even use the term for security guards, night club bouncers and an array of other greater and lesser occupations. It may surprise you that the issue of 'profession', its terminology and is titles, is often misunderstood, but understanding it is central to some of the issues surrounding nursing careers.

A profession, in the strict sense, is defined by a number of key issues. To claim that you are a professional, a member of a profession, requires certain criteria to be met. A profession should:

- provide a service to society that cannot ordinarily be carried out by all members of society (a special skill or knowledge);
- have a standard of practice or code of conduct;
- be regulated by a governing body;
- have a well-defined membership (a register of practising membership);

- have autonomy of practice;
- have a gate of entry (minimum standards to access training and education);
- have a rigorous and long training and education;
- have a career progression that requires lifelong education;
- have a unique body of knowledge;
- be rewarded with high remuneration.

If we consider the profession of medicine, it is instantly apparent that it would meet such criteria (although events in recent years have thrown challenges at the medical profession in relation to this). If we consider night club bouncers, it is probably fair to say that they do not meet these criteria (although I am keen to note that I do not want to offend any bouncers anywhere).

Now consider nursing. Nurses aspire to professional status but historically would not have met the above criteria on several points. Table 2.1 below reveals how this situation has evolved over time.

Table 2.1 Nursing as a profession

Nursing as a profession	1970	2010
Provide a service to society that cannot ordinarily be carried out by all members of society (a special skill or knowledge)	Yes	Yes
Have a standard of practice or code of conduct	No	Yes
Be regulated by a governing body	Yes	Yes
Have a well-defined membership (a register of practising membership)	No – prior to the 1979 Nurses Act the Nursing Register was lifelong – and thus did not represent a list of 'practising' nurses	A live (living and practising) Register came into place in 1980
Have autonomy of practice	No – nurses' activity was directed primarily by the medical profession	Arguably, the situation has changed, with nurses taking far more autonomous responsibility
Have a gate of entry (minimum standards to access training and education)	Yes – although nurse education was service-driven and vocational, rather than a university-based process	Yes – all graduate entry
Have a rigorous and long training and education	Yes – but not academically recognised	Yes
Have a career progression that requires lifelong education	No – there was no requirement for further education, and career progression was limited	Yes – nurses must demonstrate ongoing education, and the career structure is far more established
Have a unique body of knowledge	Not really – nursing theory was underdeveloped, and nursing research was rare	Yes – nursing is now much more clearly defined in terms of theory and evidence
Receive high remuneration	No – nurses' pay was traditionally poor	Much improved – nurses today can command good salaries

Thus, as you can see, nursing was an aspirant profession that has over the last 40 years striven to meet the criteria for greater professional acknowledgement. As such, it has done a great deal to achieve this. For nurses who seek career advancement, this is significant as they are entering a far more structured and complex 'profession' than that which existed in 1970. The qualified nurse has scope for progression not only in managerial or educational areas, but also in research and clinical practice. In 1970, there was virtually no scope for a clinical career above the level of ward sister and minimal opportunities outside the clinical and educational environment. Today, that has all changed.

But why, you may ask, is all this relevant to your future career? The answer is that in seeking a more genuine professional status, and in response to social, financial and strategic pressures, nursing has become more and more complex, a maze or web of areas of varied expertise, and much of this structure is still emerging as this book is being written.

For example, what do we mean when we refer to specialist nurses, nurse practitioners and consultant nurses – are these titles protected, are they recordable or annotated on the Nursing Register; how were these nurses prepared for these roles, and what does the public think they are? The answer is that it is all very muddled and uncertain. The ENRiP Project (Read, 1997) identified nurses in general hospitals using a bewildering array of 'titles' to identify themselves – in excess of 700 titles were noted in just three hospitals. Since then, the profession has woken up to the need for more orderly control over nursing roles and the need to identify how these roles meet service and user needs: these may then be mapped on to sensible career planning. Indeed, the NHS has seen the introduction of competency frameworks that have sought to provide guidance on roles not just within nursing, but also for all staff at all levels within the service (e.g. the KSF).

BECOMING A STAFF NURSE – MANAGING THE TRANSITION

It is interesting to note that nearly all newly qualified nurses will seek a clinical post to start their careers. This may sound obvious, as it is exceedingly unlikely to commence a nursing career in a nurse manager's role, a lecturer's role or a more advanced clinical role as all this is dependent on experience. The cliché that we all start at the bottom is true – to an extent. I say this as I have seen newly qualified nurses access a PhD programme of study and carve out a nurse researcher role, and I have seen newly qualified nurses who have achieved rapid ascension through the ranks to senior management roles. Work carried out in Scotland has looked at fast-tracking new registrants who are high achievers to rapid promotion. Thus, it is just as well not to assume that anything is or is not possible in your career.

You have probably spent a great deal of time during your training dealing with persistent change. Changing to new clinical areas, back into college, back into practice, new essays and constant submission dates. But the key point is that you were always a student, a learner. The step to being qualified nurse is different. There will be no further set study blocks or changes of clinical area in the immediate future. You are a staff nurse and you will remain in the clinical area you have chosen at least for the time being. This may be daunting, off-duty rolling out interminably in front of you, working night duty, weekends and holidays. The structured chaos of your training will change to the staff nurse routines of your first clinical area.

But it is more than just changes of routine that you will now experience. You are now a professional in your own right, and you are now bound by the requirements of the profession. That responsibility will remain with you for the rest of your career, and you could at any time break those rules and have your privilege to practise removed. I think it is well to instil a certain awareness of this in all professional nurses as we have a public trust that we cannot betray.

Despite the point that I made above on the possibilities open to new registrants, there is a school of thought that promotes the process of 'settling in', a probationer period that allows new registrants to find their feet. Indeed, the NMC is looking to make this a mandatory requirement in future. Those first few months as a qualified nurse are unique. Everything that you learnt as a student will slowly come into play. In fact, you may not at first notice any great change. But as time progresses, you will increasingly be expected to take more responsibility for the management of the patients in your care and for the teams of nurses that you work with, and eventually (dependent on your area of work) you may start taking overall responsibility for being 'in charge'. However, the idea that you can only do this within the setting of a traditional hospital ward is an old-fashioned notion. Newly qualified nurses are increasingly looking to first posts in critical care, specialist areas of care or community and primary care.

Thus, your career planning will inevitably be influenced by your first qualified clinical appointment. However, it is only fair to say that many nurses' first appointments bear no relation to where their careers eventually take them. After all, many new registrants will accept any staff post if it gets them on the first rung of the ladder. Thus, the influence of your first post may not necessarily be immediately obvious. It is in your first post that you discover yourself as a nurse, what you are good at and what is not for you; this can be a difficult discovery, as no nurse can, after all, be all-singing and all-dancing all of the time. We all bring something to the care that we give, but no one can bring everything.

MANAGING THE TRANSITION TO STAFF NURSE – JULIE DAVIES

As a newly qualified nurse, I walked onto the ward with butterflies in my stomach, wondering what each shift would bring. Always I hoped that each new shift would allow me to grow in confidence, so that I could carry out all the tasks set by the more senior nurses using the skills that I had learnt and become competent at performing while a student. Occasionally, I hoped that I would not be asked too many questions by relatives, doctors or patients – questions that I often could not answer. In addition, I realised just how many questions I had to ask simply to get through a day, and thought to myself, 'How did I ever complete my training?' However, as time went by, I discovered that the number of questions I had to ask was getting fewer.

I was lucky to receive support from two mentors assigned to me within 2 weeks of starting my employment as a qualified nurse. The Trust I work for supplied a small portfolio of competencies in relation to local Trust policies and procedures. My mentors' role is to support me and ensure that I am confident to complete these competencies. I feel very lucky to have started my career within a large Trust on a general medical ward as a fellow newly qualified nurse that I kept in touch with took a position within a nursing home and felt as though she had very little support and was working alone from a very early stage in her position.

As a student nurse nearing the end of my training, I used to look forward to the day when I could put away my textbooks and start shopping on the Internet rather than researching journals for information, support and advice about how to provide recommended nursing care. But, as a newly qualified nurse, I am still using those textbooks and researching on the Internet as not a day goes by without me having to find out more about conditions, drugs and recommended care so that I can provide the best care to my patients and pass on new information to relatives and colleagues.

As a student, I always felt that I had good organisational skills. As a nurse, I feel that organisational skills are a *necessity*, along with time management. These skills are improving every day as I grow in confidence. Part of my role, as with every qualified nurse, is to delegate to other members of staff, especially support workers. However, I find this difficult as I want to be seen as a respected team member and don't want to be seen as the 'bossy newly qualified nurse'. Every day, I am learning in my profession and discovering that I cannot do everything. I am trying hard to remember that support staff are there to assist: being respectful of their position and asking them to carry out tasks within their capability is not being bossy or demanding, it's just creating a work environment that is based on teamwork and team cooperation.

As a nurse, it is important to remember that you are the patient's advocate and that patients cannot always express their wishes, views or opinions to family, friends, doctors or other members of the multidisciplinary team. The relationship between a nurse and a patient creates a very personal, private and sensitive bond. I have discovered that, by listening to my patients and encouraging them to become active in the expression of their care and treatment needs, my own skills of diplomacy and assertiveness have improved. It is my duty and responsibility to liaise with doctors and members of the multidisciplinary team to ensure that patient care needs are met holistically.

Within my first couple of months, I acted upon a patient's request to provide him with a bowl of cereal for lunch, much to the disgust of the food hostess as she had placed a large, three-course meal in front of my patient. When I removed the tray from his table, she told me abruptly that he needed to eat his meal. I politely disagreed and said that I would rather provide my patient with what he requested. My patient was very ill, was not for any further active treatment and was deteriorating rapidly. I felt that providing him with the simple pleasures that he requested prior to passing away in the near future was being respectful. Being an assertive advocate has become easier with diplomacy.

Every day on the ward is hard work. There are always new challenges, something new to learn, and every now and then a patient can become angry or upset with the nursing staff, their family or other patients. This can be upsetting, but I always remember that patients are ill and vulnerable, and that relatives are often worried or confused. I have found my nursing career extremely worthwhile and rewarding. Every day, I become stronger and more confident in my profession, and I am proud to call myself a nurse.

I will now move on to review the different nursing roles I highlighted earlier.

THE ROLE OF THE CLINICAL MENTOR (EDUCATION AND TEACHING IN PRACTICE)

In a remarkably short time, you will find yourself no longer the brand new staff nurse. Indeed, in just a few months, you will move on to be regarded as a core member of the team, and before you know it there will be another group of new staff nurses who will regard you as the more experienced professional. Teaching and mentoring others will be a fundamental and lifelong part of your professional life. The NMC expects students to have clinical mentorship, but you should not confuse classroom teaching with clinical teaching. Teaching in the clinical area, by example, is one of the fundamental experiences that all nurses learn from. By this, I mean that the student learns more by watching good practice in action than by anything else, and consequently the clinical teacher is also acutely aware that she or he is being watched too.

Let us initially consider the terms that are commonly used to describe features of learning and teaching (Box 2.5). These terms give meaning to your prospective role as a clinical mentor. You should expect mentorship and teaching to be part of your professional portfolio. However, the two terms, although intimately linked, are not entirely the same, and in the next section I will briefly explore this difference.

Teaching

Teaching may be described as the activity of educating or instructing or teaching, an activity that imparts knowledge or skill. There are many dimensions to teaching, from formal classroom instruction through to teaching in clinical practice, and it is clinical teaching that you, as a new staff nurse, will soon come to be most familiar with. The teacher in the clinical area teaches not by formal instruction, but by example. As the more junior nurse and student joins you and observes your professional practice, they learn by observation and exposure to best practice. This is a crucial distinction, as many clinical nurses do not understand that they are teachers simply by virtue of what they do in their everyday practice.

Mentorship

Mentors may be called by many names, and many learned people will exhort at length the nuances that make these titles different (mentor, supervisor, clinical teacher and preceptor being but a few). However, for the purposes of this book, we can accept a basic and generic definition of a mentor as a wise and trusted counsellor or teacher, a person who supervises workers or the work done by others, or simply as an instructor.

You will have experienced mentorship as a student and should therefore have a fairly clear idea of what it is about. You will almost certainly have had mentors whom you favoured over others. It may help for you to think back to that: why was that, what was it about the 'good' mentors that you preferred? Essentially, mentorship in the clinical environment is founded on positive relationships and mutual respect between the mentor and the student. Mentorship is about helping students to manage their own leaning, develop their own skills and improve their performance while the mentor motivates, supports and encourages.

BOX 2.5 TEACHING AND LEARNING TERMS (ADAPTED FROM BARTON, 2009)

EDUCATION

The act or process of imparting or acquiring general knowledge, developing the powers of reasoning and judgement, and generally of preparing oneself or others intellectually for life.

TEACHING

The activity of educating or instructing or teaching; an activity that imparts knowledge or skill.

TRAINING

An activity leading to skilled behaviour.

LEARNING

The cognitive process of acquiring skill or knowledge.

Acquired behaviour.

AIM

An anticipated outcome that is intended or that guides your planned actions.

OBJECTIVE

The goal intended to be attained.

An intended learning outcome.

COMPETENCE

The condition by which a person is adequately qualified/possession of the required skill, knowledge, qualification or capacity.

A competence is a statement that describes the ability to do something adequately (regardless of the individual performing the skill).

COMPETENCY

This is a statement, often used in assessment check lists, that describes the ability to do something adequately.

CURRICULUM

An integrated course of academic and or skills-based studies.

Types of curriculum:

• Behavioural (outcome-driven – competencies)
• Experiential (learning from experience)
• Apprenticeship (guided by an expert in practice to learn skill(s)/learning an occupation in practice).

SYLLABUS

An outline of the main points of a course of study, the subjects of a course of lectures, the contents of a curriculum.

ASSESSMENT

The act of judging or assessing a person or situation or event.

Related terminology:

• Formative (developmental and/or diagnostic assessment – not usually included in the final grading)
• Summative (formal testing that produces marks and grades)
• Written assessment, portfolio assessment, observation assessment, oral assessment.

MENTOR (SUPERVISOR, CLINICAL TEACHER, PRECEPTOR)

A wise and trusted counsellor or teacher.

A person who supervises workers or the work done by others.

An instructor.

Thus, as a practice-based profession, healthcare has traditionally assumed and ensured that clinical staff support, supervise and teach students within the practice setting. This concept of mentorship is a process by which students work alongside practitioners and learn from experts in a safe, supportive and educationally conducive environment. Mentors are skilled experienced practitioners who possess good communication skills, are proficient in teaching and have a positive attitude towards facilitating and guiding students through their clinical placement and towards the successful completion of their clinical outcomes.

Assessment

You have, as a student nurse, been subject to endless assessment. Assessment is the act of judging or assessing a person, a set of skills, a situation or an event. As a qualified nurse, you will be expected to assess students, junior staff and even perhaps your peers.

Assessment is an activity that comes in many forms but may for simplicity be divided between two polarities. At one end, there is formative assessment: this is a developmental and/or diagnostic assessment and is not usually included in the final grading. In contrast, at the other end lies summative assessment, this being a formal process of testing that produces final marks and grades.

Assessment tools are extremely varied, and it is not the intention of this book to delve into the details of educational science (although you might like to read more in Sue Hinchliff's book). However, you will be familiar with such tools of assessment as written essays, written examinations, reflective accounts and perhaps clinical examinations. As a clinical mentor, you will be called on to observe students in practice, instruct them and make professional evaluations of their competence in practice.

Competence/competency

Although 'competence' and 'competency' have become well used terms in healthcare, they are often used incorrectly, with only a little thought having been given to their meaning or definition.

Competence may be simply defined as the condition by which one is adequately qualified and assessed as being in possession of the required skill and knowledge to perform a task or role. It follows that 'a *competency*' is a statement that describes the ability to do something adequately (regardless of the individual performing the skill). Finally, being '*competent*' is the observed behaviour that confirms an ability to do something adequately.

There are literally legions of competency frameworks that are used to measure and structure health professions and health professionals. You will be familiar with the NHS's KSF and the NMC's competency frameworks, and there are others that are focused on specific roles or levels of practice. These competency frameworks enable employers to judge the scope and extent of employees' activity, and ultimately to assure the public that everyone is doing what they ought to, and at the level that they ought to. They also enable staff to assess others, as they provide measurable, observable outcomes and behaviours. As a mentor, you will observe students, and you will find that eventually you will be expected to sign off competencies as achieved. To become a 'sign-off' mentor, you will be expected to undertake and complete a short course (run by your NHS employer, often in conjunction with a local university) that will give you authority to do this.

It is worth noting that not everyone is a fan of competencies. It is argued that they represent only part of the professional's practice, and that certain attributes are difficult to 'sign off'. For example, it is a matter for judgement whether a student can be deemed to be kind or caring, or to have empathy. And indeed, as a mentor, you are expected to use your professional judgement, and this will be trusted by educators and other peers.

YOUR ROLE AS A TEACHER

Reflect on your current role and note down any educational activities you are involved in. Do you teach or mentor students or others – and if so what do you teach, and how?

Do you think you are a good teacher, and how do you evaluate this? What do you think you could do to improve your teaching skills?

THE ROLE OF THE WARD SISTER/CHARGE NURSE

The term 'sister' is a historical title from the time when nurses were exclusively female nuns who were drawn from the convents. Although that era is long gone, the title 'sister' is an enduring one in the public's mind. Ward sisters and their more modern male equivalents, charge nurses, are associated with the traditional management and leadership of the hospital ward. Indeed, the strategic view of the role of the ward sister/charge nurse is one that sees them as essential to hospital nursing and pivotal in the organisation and delivery of hospital patient care. It is the ward sister/charge nurse who informs, enacts and monitors the standards of nursing care on the hospital ward, ensuring that nursing is practised within a clinical governance framework. They are responsible for running a ward (or unit) and may have some form of budgetary control. They are also responsible for a host of other management issues (e.g. staff rostering [off-duty], staff management, ward equipment and delegation of duties or tasks to mention just a few). These nurses usually attract a Band 6 or 7 salary depending on the size of the ward/department and/or whether their responsibility is shared. It is worth noting that there are also senior sisters and charge nurses, these designations relating to clinical areas where there is a need to employ several nurses at a ward manager level (e.g. in A&E). In these instances, one of these senior managers often acts as the senior ward manager. These nurses attract a pay-banding of anywhere between 6 and 8c. Such roles will be defined by a job description, and these may vary widely depending on the type of ward or unit. Nevertheless, it is possible to provide a simplified description that captures much of what would be expected of you in this role (Box 2.6).

BOX 2.6 SAMPLE JOB DESCRIPTION OF A WARD SISTER/CHARGE NURSE

The ward sister/charge nurse will:

- Demonstrate effective leadership and staff management/development
- Be clinically competent in the initial assessment of admissions and contribute to direct and evaluated patient care on a regular basis
- Use evidence-based standards to support nursing
- Lead the development of consistent and evidence-based clinical policies, protocols, procedures and audit in the clinical area
- Develop effective communication with all healthcare staff, patients and families
- Ensure record-keeping and monitor compliance with NMC standards for record-keeping
- Ensure that due regard is given to the customs, values and spiritual beliefs of patients/clients
- Be responsible for the custody, ordering and storage of all drugs within the ward/unit, according to legal requirements
- In collaboration with an educational coordinator, identify the individual learning needs of all staff through Knowledge and Skills Framework outlines and personal development reviews
- Ensure appropriate learning and provide a timely response in relation to patient concerns or complaints, implementing action plans to address any issues raised by the complainant
- Monitor and manage staff sickness/absence following employer guidelines
- Ensure that an effective clinical learning environment is developed and maintained
- Maintain accurate records of training and development and ensure staff compliance with mandatory training
- Encourage reflective practice, including ongoing professional development
- Participate in clinical supervision.

There are many issues surrounding the professional nature and organisational context of the contemporary ward sister/charge nurse role. As the profession evolves, and the nature, delivery and emphasis of healthcare changes, the nature of the ward sister/charge nurse will also inevitably change. The breadth of the role encompasses leadership and management, clinical practice, and education and teaching. Thus, ward sisters and charge nurses are constantly balancing the varied and different aspects of their job, and that job may vary according to the context of their setting and specialty. What is clear is that the role requires a significant breadth and depth of knowledge, skills and responsibility to ensure nursing standards. Key areas of that authority have been highlighted in numerous strategic policies that identify the pivotal role of the ward sister/charge nurse in such areas as ward cleanliness, infection control and nutrition.

Ward sisters/charge nurses are challenged by many of the issues that are arising from the organisation and system issues that enable modern-day hospitals to function. Today, they are faced with rapid patient turnover, shorter hospital stays, high patient throughput, higher patient dependency and consequent high levels of bed occupancy. This has resulted in, or perhaps is also a consequence of, increasingly high levels of patient acuity. That is to say, that most patients on the ward today will be acutely unwell, more so than in the past. In addition, it is also important to remember that another change that has impacted on ward sisters and charge nurses is the reorganisation of medical education. This has resulted in junior doctors no longer being attached to consultant firms and wards, and has consequently produced clinical ward teams that are different from those previously seen; this has a knock-on effect on the supervision and education provided to them by the whole multidisciplinary team.

Ward sisters and charge nurses lead clinical practice; they manage, supervise and attend to the totality of the ward environment. Ideally, they should be supernumerary to shifts numbers, freeing them to oversee standards of care from a multidisciplinary perspective, that of nurses, doctors and all members of the professional health team. This will allow them to set appropriate standards, teach clinical practice and procedures, and be a role model for good professional practice. Most importantly, they know their patients and their healthcare needs and are visible to ward visitors as the ward leader.

THE ROLE OF A DISTRICT NURSE AND GENERAL PRACTICE NURSE

We have so far focused on discussion that may be seen as being very 'acute' or 'hospital' focused. Thus, it is important now to remember that the community and primary care are a fundamental part of the care spectrum. Indeed, it is also worth noting that the Darzi themes of care are seen as transcending the traditional primary/secondary care and hospital/community divisions. Thus, that division between acute and primary care has become increasingly blurred in recent years.

The NMC sets standards and records the registration of 'Specialist Community Public Health Nurses' (SCPHNs), who practise in various service areas, for example:

- nursing in the home;
- health visiting;
- occupational health;
- school nursing;
- sexual health;
- health protection;
- family health nursing in Scotland.

The NMC has been careful not to identify specific titles in this part of the Register but instead notes the competencies and skills used when working with specific communities and addressing health inequalities and promoting public health. Thus, nurses working within this area of practice need to undertake programmes of study and assessment that will allow them to practice as a SCPHN. District nurses and general practice nurses both fall into the category of SCPHN, and both play crucial roles in the primary healthcare and community team.

Although I have chosen two roles in this section, both associated with the community and primary care, it is important to remember that they are quite distinct roles. It is also important to note that both these roles are underpinned by formal programmes of study that, on successful completion, will make you eligible to apply to be recorded on Part 1 of the NMC's professional Register as an SCPHN district nurse or SCHPN general practice nurse. Let us consider first the district nurse.

The district nurse

District nurses provide nursing care and family support to people in their homes or in residential care homes. They provide direct patient care, and work with patients and their families to enable them to care, where possible, for themselves. They see patients of all ages and with all conditions, ranging from those recently discharged from hospital or with acute illness through to those with long-term health problems and disabilities. It is perhaps to be expected that many patients seen by district nurses will be elderly. There is no question that enabling patients to stay within their own homes, to manage where possible their own care and to avoid hospital admission or readmission, is a fundamental vision of health strategy, and as such district nurses are central to that intent.

District nurses have particular skills with which to deal with their role. Entering people's houses and assessing the healthcare needs of patients and families in their own environment can be challenging, and this requires developed skills of diplomacy and tact to ensure the highest level of professional care. And of course district nurses do not have to hand all the facilities and technologies of a modern hospital, so they have to be creative and adaptable. They carry their own caseload, and will work closely with other social and health service agencies (GP practices, social services and voluntary organisations) in providing packages of care.

The general practice nurse

General practice nurses work in a health centre or in GP surgeries either as lone practitioners or as a part of a team of practitioners. They are a fundamental part of the wider multiprofessional primary healthcare team, which includes doctors, specialist and community nurses, pharmacists, and other allied health professionals (AHPs) and therapists. The general practice nurse has a varied role that may include a caseload of dealing with people who present at the surgery with acute symptoms or minor injuries, undertaking routine wound dressings, managing vaccination programmes, assisting in minor surgery, managing and monitoring health screening or family planning, and managing health promotion (e.g. smoking cessation).

Thus, the general practice nurse is in every sense of the term a generalist. They see all sorts of undifferentiated health needs, deal with a diversity of chronic health problems and manage health promotion programmes. General practice nurses, along with GPs, are the foundation of health centre primary care.

THE ROLE OF THE ADVANCED (CLINICAL) NURSE
Advanced practice explained

There is no aspect of nursing practice that has led to more discussion, debate, research, investigation and writing than that of advanced practice. This is almost certainly because, as I indicated earlier, nursing has in many ways had an underdeveloped career structure, and thus it has taken us some time to understand what advanced practice actually means. Fortunately for the new nurse today, we now have a better developed notion of what this means, and many tools at our disposal to help us. What is certainly clear is that (as we move to an all graduate pre-registration status) future advanced nurses should be studying and learning at a Masters level.

Definitions of advanced nursing practice

There are many definitions of advanced practice, and I do not intend to spend too much time reproducing these. However, for clarity, I will offer two of the most used definitions, shown in the Professional Guidelines boxes. The first is a concise definition provided by the International Council of Nurses; the second is the more wordy one offered by the NMC.

PROFESSIONAL GUIDELINES

INTERNATIONAL COUNCIL OF NURSES DEFINITION OF ADVANCED PRACTICE

A registered nurse who has acquired the expert knowledge base, complex decision-making skills and clinical competencies for expanded practice, the characteristics of which are shaped by the context and/or country in which s/he is credentialed to practice. A Master's degree is recommended for entry level.

(International Council of Nurses, 2002)

PROFESSIONAL GUIDELINES

NURSING AND MIDWIFERY COUNCIL DEFINITION OF ADVANCED PRACTICE

Advanced nurse practitioners are highly experienced and educated members of the care team who are able to diagnose and treat your healthcare needs or refer you to an appropriate specialist if needed.

Advanced nurse practitioners are highly skilled nurses who can:

- Take a comprehensive patient history
- Carry out physical examinations
- Use their expert knowledge and clinical judgement to identify the potential diagnosis
- Refer patients for investigations where appropriate
- Make a final diagnosis
- Decide on and carry out treatment, including the prescribing of medicines, or refer patients to an appropriate specialist
- Use their extensive practice experience to plan and provide skilled and competent care to meet patients' health and social care needs, involving other members of the health care team as appropriate
- Ensure the provision of continuity of care including follow-up visits
- Assess and evaluate, with patients, the effectiveness of the treatment and care provided and make changes as needed
- Work independently, although often as part of a health care team
- Provide leadership

Make sure that each patient's treatment and care is based on best practice.

(Nursing and Midwifery Council, 2006)

Having these definitions is all well and good, but it is also important that you understand one of the most fundamental concepts that underpins advanced practice. The naming of nursing roles as 'specialists', 'nurse practitioners', 'consultant nurses' and a plethora of other similar variants on these titles creates difficulties for the public, service leads and practitioners. There has been, until fairly recently, no shared understanding among stakeholders of what these titles mean, and actually entail. For example, is a clinical nurse specialist practising at the same, a higher or a lower level than a generalist nurse practitioner? Indeed, what do we mean when we refer to a specialist and a generalist (Box 2.7)?

BOX 2.7   GENERALISTS AND SPECIALISTS

THE GENERALIST

A healthcare worker/professional (doctor, nurse, support worker, physiotherapist, etc.) working with client groups that have undifferentiated or undiagnosed health needs.

THE ADVANCED GENERALIST PRACTITIONER

is commonly, but not exclusively, titled a

Nurse practitioner

THE SPECIALIST

A healthcare worker/professional (doctor, nurse, support worker, physiotherapist, etc.) working with a specific client group or a specific disease or pathology.

THE ADVANCED SPECIALIST PRACTITIONER

is commonly, but not exclusively, titled a

Clinical nurse specialist

Thus, it is increasingly recognised that the 'specialist' and 'generalist' represent opposite poles of a lateral continuum, whereas 'novice' to 'expert' forms a vertical continuum. In this model (Fig. 2.2), specialist and generalist nurses could be novices or experts. It is quite possible to have a novice in a very specialist field, or conversely a generalist who is advanced in their level of practice.

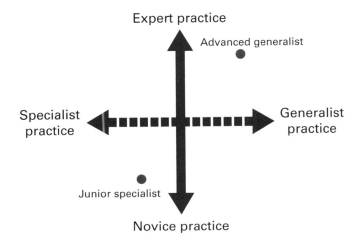

Figure 2.2 The practice cross, as described in the Advanced Nursing Practice Toolkit (NHS Scotland, 2011)

Beyond the clinical domain

You will have of course noted that, and perhaps wondered why, I put the word 'clinical' in brackets in the title of this section. The work of Modernising Nursing Careers (Department of Health, 2006) and the subsequent Advanced Practice Toolkit (Department of Health, 2010) acknowledged that there were many nurses who were working at an 'advanced' level but who may not have been working in a specifically 'clinical' role. This was crucially important, recognising that 'advanced practice' was a level of practice, rather than a specific role, and could equally encompass those working within or across many spheres of practice – in clinical, research, education and/or managerial/leadership roles.

If you look at Fig. 2.3, you will see that these spheres of practice all interact with each other, and, as indicated in the career maps earlier in this chapter, advanced nursing practice roles will almost certainly be composites of all of them, with certain features predominating.

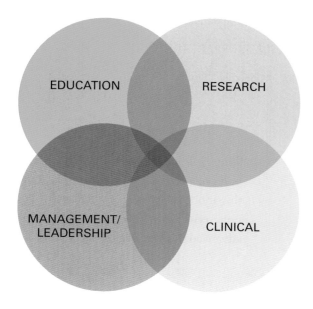

Figure 2.3 Spheres of practice, as described in the Advanced Nursing Practice Toolkit (NHS Scotland, 2011)

THE ROLE OF THE NURSE PRESCRIBER

The introduction of legislation that allows nurses to prescribe medication is one of the most significant changes in health law since the inception of the NHS. The law on 'non-medical prescribing' encompasses nurses and AHPs such as pharmacists, physiotherapists and podiatrists – and in the future may extend to other AHPs. Non-medical prescribing has had a rather long history over the past 20 years, and I do not intend to dwell here on that complexity; therefore, I will focus this section on prescribing as it applies to nurses.

Suffice it to say that there are levels of non-medical prescribing, ranging from that which allows community nurses to prescribe from a limited list of medications, through to full independent prescribing that allows the nurse to prescribe anything from the *British National Formulary* without seeking a medical signature. Whatever level you study for, it will become a formal role that will be annotated on the NMC Register, and that is a significant responsibility.

I intend to focus on the independent nurse prescriber, who undoubtedly meets the criteria of an advanced practitioner (as outlined above), and who can have significant impact on practice. The independent nurse prescriber has scope to improve patient access to medicines, cut waiting times for patients and improve treatment responses in a wide range of clinical settings in the community and in the hospital. It has led to patients having more efficient healthcare options. Indeed, it is today increasingly likely that your patients will have their care managed by advanced nurses who are prescribers, either in the GP surgery or while being treated at a hospital for physical or mental health problems. Nurse prescribers can manage a vast variety of conditions depending on their area of expertise.

Becoming an independent nurse prescriber requires the successful completion of an intense programme of education. These programmes are usually offered by the schools and colleges of health at local universities, are validated by the NMC and last about 6–9 months. Some universities include independent prescribing as a module within their advanced practice Masters-level programmes. The programmes are strictly assessed on a variety of aspects of clinical assessment, pathology, pharmacology, the law and numeracy, all applied to prescribing. They will certainly want you to have had some considerable clinical experience before being accepted onto such a programme, and you will have to show that you have the full support of your employer. In addition, the law requires that you identify a medical practitioner to support your learning and practice throughout your studies.

It must be said that, as with any other profession, the independent nurse prescriber does *not* have a free licence to prescribe any drug. The scope of professional practice clearly confines every practitioner to operate only within their area of expertise, and in addition, every employer will have protocols in place to ensure that the prescribers only practise within their area of expertise. Nevertheless, nurses who prescribe are educated and highly skilled professionals – the majority of nurses who prescribe have at least 10 years' nursing experience before starting their prescribing training.

THE ROLE OF THE NURSE MANAGER/NURSE EXECUTIVE

There is a well-known view that asks 'Why do we need leaders – surely a group of intelligent, well-educated people can get by without having to have leaders?' However, in reality, in a profession as complex as nursing, and in a health service as vast as the NHS, the simple fact is that 'someone' has to manage it all.

A nurse manager organises nursing services, wherever those may be. They manage human resources, information, clinical services, staff recruitment and budgeting. The role of a nurse manager not only contributes to today's nursing services, but also determines the requirements for the future configurations of the service. Thus, nurse managers may operate at a unit level, organising a collective of wards, hospital specialist services and community services, through to those at the most senior level – senior board executives.

Thus, nurse managers may be seen as not only service organisers, but also strategic leaders of the nursing profession, with responsibility for nursing staff and for the management and the delivery of nursing care. In addition (depending on the specifics of their role), they have responsibility for professional development, education and clinical governance.

Today, it is usual for NHS organisations to have an executive nurse as a board member, with a well-defined structure of assistant executives who manage and control the delivery of nursing services. These nurse executives influence decision-making at the highest level, safeguarding nursing resources. These most senior nurses have to develop business skills while also retaining their focus on the fundamentals of patient care. Such senior roles are naturally well remunerated, with salaries ranging from Band 8a through to Band 9.

This may seem all very grand and out of your reach at this time. But the simple fact of the matter is that some of you who read this book will advance your careers to senior nursing management. This may take time and a great deal of effort, but one thing is certain – the profession requires future leaders.

THE ROLE OF THE NURSE EDUCATOR

Earlier in this chapter, I discussed the role of clinical mentorship that you will all assume in the early part of your clinical career. As a result of this experience, many nurses find that they enjoy teaching students and imparting knowledge to the next generation of professionals, ensuring that the next generation of nurses are competent and confident in the practice setting.

It follows that some will eventually seek to develop their careers in nurse education as a lecturer in nursing. If that is the case, many will start by getting involved with the local university, undertaking occasional teaching sessions that are often related to their area of specialist clinical skill. Many health service organisations will have some staff who are appointed as lecturer practitioners – working part of their time in the university and part of their time in practice. This is beneficial to everyone as the university reaps the benefit of a practising and experienced nurse, while the health service nurtures a practitioner with skills in education.

Being appointed as a full-time lecturer will require some professional and academic requirements. First, you will need to be on an appropriate part of the NMC's professional Register, and you will have to have worked in areas where students were gaining practical experience. Today, most universities would expect applicants to have a Masters level qualification, or at the very least be working towards this while in post. If you have developed skills in a particular clinical specialty, undertaken study in a particular area of professional practice or undertaken study or research, these will certainly improve your chances on application. If appointed, you will be required to take a postgraduate certificate in learning and teaching (higher education) – in other words, teacher training. These training programmes are designed to be undertaken alongside your lecturing work.

Lecturers in nursing are varyingly responsible for the delivery of both pre- and post-registration/undergraduate and postgraduate teaching in universities (depending on their experience, specialty and type of contract). They plan educational programmes, manage their delivery, teach on them, evaluate them and provide support and direction for their students. They will also maintain significant links with the clinical areas that their students are attending, and ensure that these areas are offering an appropriate environment for learning.

As university employees, lecturers in nursing are subject to the career and pay framework that exists within higher education, and the remuneration for this is usually very favourable – ranging from the equivalent of a Band 8 to a Band 9 salary. They will be expected to undertake some research and to be publishing work in journals or writing chapters in textbooks. They should be the experts of the nursing profession from a knowledge perspective, imparting the fundamental skills and expanding the evidence that underpins modern nursing practice. Today, many full-time lecturers progress eventually to undertake a PhD or a professional doctorate and may become senior lecturers, readers or professors. Nevertheless, remaining clinically credible and competent is crucial, and most lecturers combine their academic and teaching role with some form of work in a clinical setting.

THE ROLE OF THE NURSE RESEARCHER

Nursing is an evidence-based profession, and it follows that the majority of such evidence must be developed through research. As professional nurses, we must all ask questions and think critically about our practice, ensure that it is valid and reliable, and be able to access and critique evidence before it is implemented. Indeed, the skills of critique are a fundamental part of pre-registration undergraduate curricula. However, there need to be nurses whose skills are those of research itself. Such individuals will often naturally rise from the ranks of lecturers, but I have known many well-regarded researchers who have risen from the ranks of clinical nurses. There is considerable encouragement for this.

In the most basic sense, nurse researchers set sensible research questions to advance nursing knowledge and practice, and collect data in order to answer these questions. They review and analyse those data and disseminate the results via publications and conferences in order to inform and change practice. This is, of course, a gross oversimplification. Researchers will have methodologies and research methods that they specialise in, and they will apply these in the context of their clinical interests. Nursing research may range from large-scale quantitative statistical studies through to exploratory qualitative studies that explore aspects of the human experience. Studies may be supported by substantial grants and have a team of researchers, or may be small-scale projects with single researchers.

It is perhaps unsurprising that nurse researchers are often employed by, or at the very least closely connected with, universities. Such roles are crucially important to the future of nursing, but they are highly specialist and will require many years of experience, as well as a clear determination to undertake research through a process of advanced education. For the career nurse researcher, a first aspiration must be a PhD.

THE ROLE OF THE NURSE CONSULTANT

Nurse consultant posts were first established in the UK in the late 1990s by the Labour government of that time and were seen as central to health service modernisation. Since their inception, they have progressed to become an established role in the profession. Nurse consultants provide the nursing profession with a career pinnacle, arguably one of the most significant and influential roles within the profession. While they spend a minimum of 50 per cent of their time working directly with patients, they also carry a range of different responsibilities that may involve consultancy on local and healthcare policy, budgetary control, undertaking research and publishing, and providing strategic leadership. In addition, nurse consultants are expected to be involved in and contributing to nurse education, training and development.

Nevertheless, each and every nurse consultant's role will be very different, depending upon the area of practice, the needs of the employer, and local and regional issues. But it cannot be understated that nurses working at this level are among the highest paid of their profession and usually secure such posts following long careers with considerable experience, seniority and high levels of advanced education. A number of nurse consultants are authors of chapters in the second section of this book – you will be able to read more about their careers there.

Conclusion

This chapter set out to explore the scope of nursing roles, and possible career pathways, in the modern nursing profession. If you have read this far, you will have seen that the profession offers a huge range of diverse options. Some may say that none of these roles appeals to them – and that they simply want to remain as caring professional bedside nurses. To that end, I would say that that in itself is the right option for many – and it is clear that we need lifelong bedside nurses to ensure that the highest level of expert nursing care is given to patients. But we are a diverse profession, and everyone in the profession brings something that we need, be they a consultant nurse, lecturer in nursing, nurse manager, ward sister, specialist, generalist or prescriber. The whole of the profession is greater than the sum of its parts, and whatever your career choice is, it will form a crucial part of a greater whole.

References

Barton TD (2009) How to assess teaching and learning. In: *The Practitioner as Teacher*, Hinchliff SM (ed.). London: Elsevier, Chapter 5.

Department of Health (2004a) *Agenda for Change*. London: HMSO.

Department of Health (2004b) *The NHS Knowledge and Skills Framework (NHS KSF) and the Development Review Process*. London: HMSO.

Department of Health (2006) *Modernising Nursing Careers – Setting the Direction*. London: HMSO.

Department of Health (2008) *A High Quality Workforce – NHS Next Stage Review* (the Darzi Report). London: HMSO.

Department of Health (2010) The Advanced Nursing Practice Toolkit. Retrieved from: http://www.advancedpractice.scot.nhs.uk (accessed November 2010).

Hinchliff SM (2009) *The Practitioner as Teacher*. London: Churchill Livingstone.

International Council of Nurses (2002) Editorial: ICN announces its position on advanced nursing roles. *International Nursing Review* 49(4): 202.

NHS Scotland (2011) Advanced Nursing Practice Toolkit. Retrieved from: http://www.advancedpractice.scot.nhs.uk/home.aspx (accessed May 2011).

Nursing and Midwifery Council (2006) The Proposed Framework for the Standard for Post-registration Nursing. Retrieved from: http://www.nmc-uk.org/Get-involved/Consultations/Past-consultations/By-year/The-proposed-framework-for-the-standard-for-post-registration-nursing---February-2005/ (accessed 17 June 2011).

Nursing and Midwifery Council (2008a) Statistical Analysis of the Register – 1 April 2007 to 31 March 2008. Retrieved from: http://www.nmc-uk.org/ (accessed October 2010).

Nursing and Midwifery Council (2008b) A Review of Pre-registration Nursing Education – Report of Consultation Findings. Retrieved from: http://www.nmc-uk.org/ (accessed October 2010).

Nursing and Midwifery Council (2010) The Prep Handbook. Retrieved from: http://www.nmc-uk.org/ (accessed October 2010).

Read, S. (1997) *Exploring New Roles in Practice: Implications of developments within the clinical team (ENRiP)*. Sheffield: DOH's Human Resources and Effectiveness Initiative, Sheffield University School of Health and Related Research.

Royal College of Nursing (2010) Royal College Review of Nursing: Pay Rates 2010/11. Retrieved from: http://www.rcn.org.uk/support/pay_and_conditions/pay_rates_2010-2011 (accessed November 2010).

Welsh Assembly Government (2008) *Post Registration Careers Framework in Wales*. Cardiff: WAG.

Chapter 3

DEVELOPING SKILLED PROFESSIONAL PRACTICE

Andrée le May

LEARNING OUTCOMES

You will learn the following from this chapter:
- **How people and organisations see nurses and nursing differently**
- **How to develop skilled professional practice**
- **How important it is to focus on the care that you give patients/service users *and* on the environment within which that care is delivered**
- **How expert practice can be constructed and delivered**

OVERVIEW

Judy Uren, the former Federal Secretary of the Australian Nursing Federation, explained that if she were to choose her career again, she would always choose nursing, 'Because it is the most exciting, diverse, frustrating, challenging, demanding career anyone could wish for. What other career allows you, in fact invites you, to be part of the intimate tapestry of life, present at the beginning of life and often there at the end of life, with a continuing role to play throughout the life-cycle?' (Maslin, 1999, p. 134). Chapter 2 gave you an inkling of this potential, and in this chapter and Chapter 4, I will try to get behind that excitement and lay out for you the components of skilled professional practice – many of which will be developed, in relation to particular domains of adult nursing, in Part Two of this book. These aspects revolve around skilled nursing practice, leadership, research utilisation, personal development and the development of others.

The first section of this chapter is about nursing – how it is defined, how it is perceived and how it is experienced by patients/services users. The second section identifies the components of skilled nursing practice as described by the Nursing and Midwifery Council (2010), while the third section moves towards an understanding of how all of these components of dignified care are integrated into expert nursing practice and the creation of person-centred workplaces (Manley et al., 2009). Throughout the chapter, you will glimpse some of the ingredients of clinical leadership and research utilisation, essential components of skilled professional practice. These strands, together with personal development and the development of others, will be discussed further in Chapter 4 and applied to specific areas of nursing practice in Part Two of the book.

About the author

I started my nursing career in 1978 as a student at Chelsea College (now King's College London) where I studied for a degree in Nursing with registration as a Registered General Nurse – most of the practical work for this was done at Charing Cross Hospital in London. Here I discovered two things – the importance of communication (verbal and non-verbal) in providing high quality, dignified, individualised care, and that research was exciting! After graduating I worked in the community in east and west London as a school nurse and family planning nurse and somewhat strangely given those two specialties, developed an affinity for caring for older people. After a couple of years I wondered which way to take my career – either train as a District Nurse or do my PhD and continue to develop my research skills. Both options got funding and I struggled to decide, eventually choosing to continue with my research journey. (I always intended to go back to the community but I never managed to!) My PhD focused on how nurses used touch when caring for older people in hospitals and long-term care wards. After my PhD studies finished I worked as a specialist nurse for research and development, charged primarily with the exciting (and daunting) task of getting nurses and midwives to use more research in their practice. This was a brilliant job which combined my passion for high quality practice with the challenges of persuading people to change the way they worked. After four years I started to think about teaching nursing and I left the NHS for the higher education sector where as a lecturer I found I could combine all the things that interested me – teaching other people and helping them to develop their knowledge, researching practice in order to improve it, delivering care alongside students as they developed their skills, confidence and enthusiasm and working with qualified practitioners to improve services and care. What more could I have asked for? Nothing… so I settled into life in a university environment where close links to practice were essential and moved from lecturer to senior lecturer to reader and finally to professor. Twenty-odd years on I work part-time at the university supervising research students – the rest of my work time is taken up with service development projects in the UK and abroad, and writing, but I'm just beginning to wonder if there's still a chance to squeeze in a bit of that community nursing I missed all those years ago!

Defining nursing

You will already be familiar with the many texts that discuss the nature of nursing – it is not my intention to enter into that here – but what I would like to do is to get you to pause for a moment and think about what different groups of people perceive nursing to be.

THINKING ABOUT NURSING

In order to help you think about nursing, ask several people, from a variety of age groups, what they think nursing is and what skills they would like a nurse to have if they required nursing care. Jot their thoughts down and add yours, putting yourself, first, in the position of being a patient, and second, that of a nurse. When you are thinking about your views, try to remember what you thought before you started your nursing course and compare that to what you think now.

Now compare your jottings with the definition of nursing given by the Royal College of Nursing in the text. How similar are they? How different are they? Has hearing others' thoughts on nursing changed yours, and if so, how? And why?

Once you've thought about these questions, keep your jottings so that you can compare the components of skilled nursing practice that you have now listed with some of the views presented throughout this chapter.

Nursing is defined by the Royal College of Nursing (RCN, 2003, p.3) as 'the use of clinical judgement in the provision of care to enable people to improve, maintain or recover health, to cope with health problems, and to achieve the best possible quality of life, whatever their disease or disability until death'. This definition was recently augmented by the publication of the RCN's (2010) eight 'principles of nursing practice' in November 2010 (see the Professional Guidelines box). The principles set out what people (patients, the public and colleagues) can expect from nursing: they were co-created with patient advocate groups, nurses and partners from the Nursing and Midwifery Council (NMC) and the Department of Health and apply to all nursing settings and nursing teams (Registered Nurses, students and healthcare assistants). Launching the principles, Peter Carter, the RCN Chief Executive and General Secretary, emphasised their uniqueness in:

> [bringing] together in one place for the public what can be expected from nursing. They are designed to help patients and carers, nursing staff, employers and decision-makers know exactly what quality nursing care looks like. They clearly show good nursing practice should be underpinned by dignity, responsibility, vigilance about risk and patient involvement in their care. (Royal College of Nursing, 2003)

Add all of this information to what you have already read in Chapter 2 about the Adult Nursing field being 'immensely diverse … [demanding] skills of caring, communication, management, sensitivity, counselling, teaching and above all compassion and professionalism' and you begin to get a picture of the richness of nursing and the

PRINCIPLES OF NURSING PRACTICE

The principles are:

A: Nurses and nursing staff treat everyone in their care with dignity and humanity – they understand their individual needs, show compassion and sensitivity, and provide care in a way that respects all people equally.

B: Nurses and nursing staff take responsibility for the care they provide and answer for their own judgements and actions – they carry out these actions in a way that is agreed with their patients, and the families and carers of their patients, and in a way that meets the requirements of their professional bodies and the law.

C: Nurses and nursing staff manage risk, are vigilant about risk, and help to keep everyone safe in the places they receive health care.

D: Nurses and nursing staff provide and promote care that puts people at the centre, involves patients, service users, their families and their carers in decisions and helps them make informed choices about their treatment and care.

E: Nurses and nursing staff are at the heart of the communication process: they assess, record and report on treatment and care, handle information sensitively and confidentially, deal with complaints effectively, and are conscientious in reporting the things they are concerned about.

F: Nurses and nursing staff have up-to-date knowledge and skills, and use these with intelligence, insight and understanding in line with the needs of each individual in their care.

G: Nurses and nursing staff work closely with their own team and with other professionals, making sure patients' care and treatment is co-ordinated, is of a high standard and has the best possible outcome.

H: Nurses and nursing staff lead by example, develop themselves and other staff, and influence the way care is given in a manner that is open and responds to individual needs.

(Royal College of Nursing, 2010)

complexity of skilled professional practice. Your experiences so far will have confirmed this, as well as highlighting the importance of caring, in a dignified way, for the whole person (Turner, 2007), thereby emphasising the centrality of the patient to your professional practice.

Despite having a contemporary definition of nursing to work with (Royal College of Nursing, 2003), a set of principles for nursing practice (Royal College of Nursing, 2010) and a clear Code of Conduct (Nursing and Midwifery Council, 2008) to drive practice, many nurses would argue that these only just scratch the surface of nursing and do not capture its complexity.

THE CODE: STANDARDS OF CONDUCT, PERFORMANCE AND ETHICS FOR NURSES AND MIDWIVES (NURSING AND MIDWIFERY COUNCIL, 2008)

The people in your care must be able to trust you with their health and wellbeing. To justify that trust, you must:

- make the care of people your first concern, treating them as individuals and respecting their dignity
- work with others to protect and promote the health and wellbeing of those in your care, their families and carers, and the wider community
- provide a high standard of practice and care at all times
- be open and honest, act with integrity and uphold the reputation of your profession.

As a professional, you are personally accountable for actions and omissions in your practice and must always be able to justify your decisions. You must always act lawfully, whether those laws relate to your professional practice or personal life. Failure to comply with this code may bring your fitness to practise into question and endanger your registration. This code should be considered together with the Nursing and Midwifery Council's rules, standards, guidance and advice available from www.nmc-uk.org.

Make the care of people your first concern, treating them as individuals and respecting their dignity

Treat people as individuals
- You must treat people as individuals and respect their dignity
- You must not discriminate in any way against those in your care
- You must treat people kindly and considerately
- You must act as an advocate for those in your care, helping them to access relevant health and social care, information and support

Respect people's confidentiality
- You must respect people's right to confidentiality
- You must ensure people are informed about how and why information is shared by those who will be providing their care
- You must disclose information if you believe someone may be at risk of harm, in line with the law of the country in which you are practising

Collaborate with those in your care
- You must listen to the people in your care and respond to their concerns and preferences
- You must support people in caring for themselves to improve and maintain their health
- You must recognise and respect the contribution that people make to their own care and wellbeing
- You must make arrangements to meet people's language and communication needs
- You must share with people, in a way they can understand, the information they want or need to know about their health

Ensure you gain consent
- You must ensure that you gain consent before you begin any treatment or care
- You must respect and support people's rights to accept or decline treatment and care
- You must uphold people's rights to be fully involved in decisions about their care
- You must be aware of the legislation regarding mental capacity, ensuring that people who lack capacity remain at the centre of decision making and are fully safeguarded
- You must be able to demonstrate that you have acted in someone's best interests if you have provided care in an emergency

Maintain clear professional boundaries

- You must refuse any gifts, favours or hospitality that might be interpreted as an attempt to gain preferential treatment
- You must not ask for or accept loans from anyone in your care or anyone close to them
- You must establish and actively maintain clear sexual boundaries at all times with people in your care, their families and carers

Work with others to protect and promote the health and wellbeing of those in your care, their families and carers, and the wider community

Share information with your colleagues

- You must keep your colleagues informed when you are sharing the care of others
- You must work with colleagues to monitor the quality of your work and maintain the safety of those in your care
- You must facilitate students and others to develop their competence

Work effectively as part of a team

- You must work cooperatively within teams and respect the skills, expertise and contributions of your colleagues
- You must be willing to share your skills and experience for the benefit of your colleagues
- You must consult and take advice from colleagues when appropriate
- You must treat your colleagues fairly and without discrimination
- You must make a referral to another practitioner when it is in the best interests of someone in your care

Delegate effectively

- You must establish that anyone you delegate to is able to carry out your instructions
- You must confirm that the outcome of any delegated task meets required standards
- You must make sure that everyone you are responsible for is supervised and supported

Manage risk

- You must act without delay if you believe that you, a colleague or anyone else may be putting someone at risk
- You must inform someone in authority if you experience problems that prevent you working within this code or other nationally agreed standards
- You must report your concerns in writing if problems in the environment of care are putting people at risk

Provide a high standard of practice and care at all times

Use the best available evidence

- You must deliver care based on the best available evidence or best practice
- You must ensure any advice you give is evidence based if you are suggesting healthcare products or services
- You must ensure that the use of complementary or alternative therapies is safe and in the best interests of those in your care

Keep your skills and knowledge up to date

- You must have the knowledge and skills for safe and effective practice when working without direct supervision
- You must recognise and work within the limits of your competence
- You must keep your knowledge and skills up to date throughout your working life
- You must take part in appropriate learning and practice activities that maintain and develop your competence and performance

Keep clear and accurate records

Record keeping: Guidance for nurses and midwives
- You must keep clear and accurate records of the discussions you have, the assessments you make, the treatment and medicines you give and how effective these have been
- You must complete records as soon as possible after an event has occurred
- You must not tamper with original records in any way
- You must ensure any entries you make in someone's paper records are clearly and legibly signed, dated and timed
- You must ensure any entries you make in someone's electronic records are clearly attributable to you
- You must ensure all records are kept securely

Be open and honest, act with integrity and uphold the reputation of your profession

Act with integrity
- You must demonstrate a personal and professional commitment to equality and diversity
- You must adhere to the laws of the country in which you are practising
- You must inform the NMC if you have been cautioned, charged or found guilty of a criminal offence
- You must inform any employers you work for if your fitness to practise is called into question

Deal with problems
- You must give a constructive and honest response to anyone who complains about the care they have received
- You must not allow someone's complaint to prejudice the care you provide for them
- You must act immediately to put matters right if someone in your care has suffered harm for any reason
- You must explain fully and promptly to the person affected what has happened and the likely effects
- You must cooperate with internal and external investigations

Be impartial
- You must not abuse your privileged position for your own ends
- You must ensure that your professional judgement is not influenced by any commercial considerations

Uphold the reputation of your profession
- You must not use your professional status to promote causes that are not related to health
- You must cooperate with the media only when you can confidently protect the confidential information and dignity of those in your care
- You must uphold the reputation of your profession at all times

(Nursing and Midwifery Council, 2008, pp. 1–8)

In an attempt to capture this complexity – the richness of nursing – I reviewed a collection of 50 interviews with nursing and midwifery leaders from all parts of the world (Maslin, 1999); the interviewees talked about their varied nursing careers and, by doing this, exposed the richness of nursing itself at the end of the last millennium. In order to gain a more contemporary view, I compared their comments with the most up-to-date viewpoint on nursing practice in the UK – the report of the former Prime Minister's commission on nursing and midwifery (Keen, 2010) and some information about what the public and patients think about nurses. Finally, I reviewed the most recent and influential regulatory information available to direct nursing practice, and the bedrock of undergraduate nursing curricula in the UK – the NMC standards (Nursing and Midwifery Council, 2010). All of this then became the core information that I drew on in order to write the next two sections of this chapter.

Melding all of these sets of information together and comparing them with my own reflections on my career as a practitioner, teacher and researcher made me look for a way to show how important they are *collectively* to the notion of expert practice – the type of practice that you, in fact we all, aspire to; I will pay more attention to this at the end of the chapter.

WHAT NURSES SAY ABOUT NURSING

The RCN's principles of nursing practice are very specific and clearly articulate what is expected of each nurse and the broader team of registered nurses, students and support workers. Their principles also echo some of the thoughts from nurse leaders at the beginning of the millennium (Box 3.1) and those of a decade later, expressed through the views voiced in the Commission on the future of nursing and midwifery (Box 3.2).

BOX 3.1 THOUGHTS ON NURSING FROM NURSE LEADERS AROUND THE WORLD (MASLIN, 1999)

'If we achieve a single-level education we can then aim to produce nurse graduates who are committed to excellence in nursing, committed to health promotion, who are in possession of a range of specialist skills, have advanced knowledge and commitment and who will deal with each patient as a whole – mind, body and spirit – rather than simplistically applying a medical model … Nurses and midwives should use resources efficiently. They should be catalysts for change in the healthcare system by conducting research, assessing client needs, sharing in the designing of new services and developing nursing and midwifery strategies to meet these needs.' (Egypt; pp. 63–4)

'The relationship of trust … underpins all nurses' work, in whatever setting.' (UK; p. 35)

'Patients don't just want to be "cured" any more, they also want a relationship with a health professional who offers time, attention and a holistic approach to care. These qualities seem to me to be at the heart of nursing. Nursing is now – and will be more than ever in the future – not just a collection of tasks that anyone with a little training can perform at an acceptable level of competence.' (UK; p. 36)

'Caring for humanity and striving for social justice.' (Denmark; p. 28)

'[facilitation] where individuals, families and communities are empowered to take care of themselves. … Nurses should demonstrate unity, responsibility, respect for human dignity, faith, love, self-respect and self-determination.' (Switzerland: pp. 37–8)

'Nurses are healers.' (USA; p. 87)

'Nurses have a strong humanitarian value base and an altruistic desire to serve others, often subordinating their own need to those of their patients.' (World Health Organization; p. 105)

'it is the only profession that focuses uniquely on the human being as a whole and its individual possibilities to take care of its own health.' (The Netherlands; p. 137)

The Commission collected vast quantities of evidence from the professions of nursing and midwifery, patients and the public in order to establish the 'competencies, skills and support that frontline nurses and midwives need to take a central role in the design and delivery of 21st century services for those that are sick and to promote health and wellbeing' (Keen, 2010, p. 2). The commission was particularly interested in finding out what hindered the workings of the crucial role that ward sisters/charge nurses/community team leaders play and the potential for nurses and midwives to lead and manage their own services (p. 2). Box 3.2 summarises some of the thoughts produced by the Commission.

BOX 3.2 THOUGHTS ON NURSING FROM THE FORMER PRIME MINISTER'S COMMISSION ON THE FUTURE OF NURSING AND MIDWIFERY IN ENGLAND (KEEN, 2010)

Nurses are 'ideally placed to improve the experiences of service users and families, and they influence health in a wide range of health, social care and community settings. In the last decade nurses have acquired greater responsibility as autonomous and interdependent practitioners: they lead programmes of care, act as partners and employers in general practice, and also lead their own services and run their own clinics. Many are specialists who can prescribe medicines and treatments, and make referrals to other health and social care professionals.' (p. 14)

The commission reported a **six dimension** vision revealing the core of twenty-first century nursing together with twenty high level recommendations needed for the vision to become a reality. The essence of each dimension is captured below:

High quality, compassionate care with nurses delivering and coordinating physical and psychosocial care for every service user, family and carer throughout their care pathway. Promoting **health and well-being** with nurses and midwives playing important roles in health promotion, disease prevention and maintaining health and well-being – both thinking and acting health. **Caring for people with long-term conditions** through playing a recognised pivotal role in the care and support of people with long-term conditions. This will mean leading, coordinating and delivering care, helping service users to minimise the impact of their condition, manage their own care, avoid further health problems and achieve the best possible quality of life. **Promoting innovation in nursing and midwifery** by working in new ways and sometimes in new roles in response to service users' needs. **Leading services** as confident and effective leaders and champions of care, with a powerful voice at all levels of the health system. **Nursing and Midwifery** will be perceived as professions that offer worthwhile, engaging **careers** with high levels of responsibility and autonomy and opportunities for personal and professional development and fulfillment.

How does the six-dimension vision in Box 3.2 fit with the thoughts you jotted down when you had completed the activity at the start of the chapter, and with your experiences of nursing? We'll take some of these dimensions further in Chapter 4, and you will also see them returning in the chapters in Part Two.

WHAT THE PUBLIC SAYS

Intricately linked to the ways in which nurses and their regulatory and professional bodies see nursing is the public's view of nurses and nursing. The Commission, drawing on surveys from across the UK, states that the public image of nursing is out of date and that a new story of nursing needs to be told if the profession is to 'recruit suitable talent and demonstrate that nurses are not poorly educated handmaidens to doctors' (Keen, 2010, p. 4). The extract below tells us very clearly why they came to this conclusion.

Nursing retains an inherited image which belongs to the late 19th century. The lady with the lamp, the ministering angel and similar visions linger in the mind. The Briggs report reached this conclusion in 1972: nearly 40 years on, has the public image of nursing changed? The 19th-century handmaiden still flits through the minds of many members of the public. Several studies conducted in 2008–2009 on behalf of the Department of Health, NHS Education Scotland, and the NHS strategic health authorities of London, West Midlands, and Yorkshire and the Humber tell a similar story – and make sobering reading.

This extensive research reveals widespread ignorance and a host of misperceptions, based on an outdated stereotype that is at best old-fashioned and at worst condescending. It positions nursing as downtrodden. Nurses are loved but not respected, and seen as victims of their vocation, without autonomy or authority. It is nasty, poorly paid, menial work that requires empathy but not expertise. The stereotypical nurse is overworked, underpaid, stoic, put-upon, passive and unambitious. She is also female – nursing is 'reserved for women'. Typical comments included the following. 'A nurse is an assistant to the doctor – it's like a lower version of a doctor,' said a 15-year-old boy. 'I'd equate nursing with something like hairdressing; there are some skills involved but not too technical,' said a career adviser. A teacher thought nursing was 'generally not for those who want or could do a degree.' Parents said, 'I'm not sure you need to be a leader to be a good nurse... surely doctors have the final say anyway?' Both the public and nurses felt that nursing's reputation had been adversely affected by the media – 'bad things are publicized, good things are expected.' As a result, they said, all nurses needed to work to maintain public respect and confidence. Nurses themselves were unhappy with their public image. They thought they were seen as subservient and poorly skilled, and that standards were thought to be declining – views that they feared might become self-fulfilling prophecies. These misperceptions undermine morale: even though nurses mostly felt their work was positive, rewarding and fulfilling, they found their public image negative, de-energizing and demoralizing.

The discrepancy between image and reality is also likely to affect recruitment. As Briggs put it, 'the familiar association of the nurse with pain, suffering and death and the tendency to place her (almost always 'her' rather than 'him') within the setting of a hospital impedes an understanding of the great variety of jobs nurses actually do. (Committee on Nursing, 1972)

As NHS London concludes, there is a need to attract the right people to become nurses in order to maintain and promote high quality care; support and motivate current nurses; and encourage and enhance positive perceptions among other professionals, decision-makers and the public. (Keen, 2010, p. 95)

To find out more about the public image of nurses and nursing, I turned to online site YouTube (http://www.youtube.com/watch?v=Jds1AlKzVGg) and found a Canadian clip, 'Images of Nursing: "I'm just a nurse"'; much of the clip supports these findings. Watch this clip and think a little more about nursing's image and what might be needed to change it.

THINKING ABOUT NURSING – REFLECTING ON NURSING

Watch the YouTube clip 'Images of Nursing: "I'm just a nurse"' at http://www.youtube.com/watch?v=Jds1AlKzVGg . Now compare your jottings from the first 'Thinking about nursing' activity at the start of this chapter with the stereotypical images of nursing portrayed in the YouTube clip and the extract above from the Prime Minister's Commission.

Do you agree with the thoughts expressed in the YouTube clip and by the Commission? If not, why do you think there are such differing views from your own? If so, what can you and your colleagues do to change them? What skills would nurses need to develop to change these images?

Thinking about the image that people, rightly or wrongly, have of nursing is important because these sorts of perception vividly colour the public's view of nursing and may therefore impact on how people react to you (and you to them) when you are working with them as patients, services users and carers.

WHAT PATIENTS SAY

The importance of patient-centred care has long been reflected in the professional standards underpinning nursing and successive governments' healthcare policies. Over the past 20 years, these policies have emphasised not only the importance of the patient to the successful management of their illness (the best known of these probably being the Expert Patient Programme), but also the value that knowing patients' views has for the improvement of care and the achievement of organisational goals in order to create a health service 'with decisions made in partnership with clinicians, rather than by clinicians alone' (Department of Health, 2010, p. 13).

To complete this section I decided to get a more 'patient-centred' view so I looked at Healthtalkonline (http://www.healthtalkonline.org/). This website lets you read or hear more than 2000 people's experiences of health and illness. You can watch videos of interviews with people, read about others' experiences and find reliable information about conditions, treatment choices and support. There I found a very different picture from the one portrayed in the YouTube clip and in the extract from the Commission's report – a view from people experiencing nursing. In order to present a more balanced picture of nursing, I have extracted from Healthtalkonline some illustrations of what nursing has meant to a range of people with different health and illness concerns (Boxes 3.3–3.6). These quotes portrayed for me a better reality of practice.

Reading what patients have said about nurses and nursing sets the backdrop for us now to begin thinking about the components of skilled practice. All of the people in the examples experienced this, and they all experienced it in an individual way – a way that was right for each of them. Nursing individuals individually is central to the delivery of skilled dignified nursing care, and we need to think how this was possible.

BOX 3.3   THE NURSES ALWAYS HAD PLENTY OF TIME TO TALK

An extract from an interview with a 61-year-old woman who has had Parkinson's disease for 20 years. She used to work as a teacher, is married and has four children:

I honestly think that neurology centre was very good, is good. I think the nurses are good but the hospice is quite a different experience altogether because they are much more laid back and they've always got time for you. Any time. As much time as you like. Just talking and I like that. And there is one particular girl on nights and she did six nights when I was there and I really got to know her. She stated that she was going to do this, that and the other. She just explained to me what she thought she would do and if I didn't want to do anything I didn't have to do it.

(http://www.healthtalkonline.org/Dying_and_bereavement/Living_with_Dying/People/Interview/244/Category/53/Clip/3143/nurses#nurses)

BOX 3.4   A MAN DISCUSSING HIS PAIN CONTROL AND NURSING CARE AFTER AN EXTRAPLEURAL PNEUMONECTOMY

An extract from an interview with a 54-year-old man. He is married with one child and works as an engineer in a nuclear power station:

The epidural stayed I think five days but that was my choice when to have it out. … after the first day they took my chest drain out and [it] just seemed, each day they could get rid of a few tubes or wires so that each day was better. On the second day after my operation they actually had me up and walking around the ward, albeit with nurses holding the drips and things like that. And again I didn't feel too bad but I presume it's because I had an epidural, other pain killers, and so you know lots of drugs. But I was certainly quite lucid; I didn't feel as zonked out or anything like that, I felt as if I knew what was going on. The nurses were really good. In the high dependency unit I had my own nurse twenty-four hours a day.

(http://www.healthtalkonline.org/Cancer/Lung_Cancer/People/Interview/193/Category/83/Clip/1778/nurses#nurses)

BOX 3.5   THE HEART FAILURE SPECIALIST NURSE

An extract from an interview with a 49-year-old man with heart failure. He is married with three children and unemployed. He has been ill for 5 years, experiencing frequent episodes of chest pain and breathlessness. He believes that the visits he receives from the heart failure specialist nurse have kept him out of hospital for the last 2 years:

The nurse that comes out just now, she'll come out and take my bloods and the IMR – take them back to the hospital. She's usually here about 10 o'clock in the morning, and by 4 o'clock I've got the results from the hospital, blood test results; she phones me up that day and tells me everything's fine, or if I'm a wee bit off she usually speaks to the consultant as well at the time, and he'll say well you know put the water tablets up or cut them back, try something else.

But basically the system I think is fantastic. It's kept me out of hospital a year, maybe two years, I think, yeah, two years now. I've been in a few times when they take you in for a test or something.

One day I went up to the hospital for my tests, my drug test at the clinic; and found my blood pressure was sky high and so they took me in for 24 hours; didn't find a reason for it, it was just one of these things. Between the drug tests and the cardiac nurse, I think there's a great system. I think every hospital should have one and a lot of hospitals don't have it.

(http://www.healthtalkonline.org/heart_disease/Heart_Failure/Topic/1799/Interview/557/Clip/2288/)

BOX 3.6 THE OUTREACH NURSES

An extract from an interview with a 35-year-old woman who was admitted to intensive care because of pneumonia and developed septicaemia. She spent 3 weeks in ICU, 36 hours in a high-dependency unit and 5 weeks on a general ward. She is married with two children:

> And then on the sort of second morning of being in step down I kind of had what they call, I can't remember the phrase now, what they call, outreach nurses, come and talk to me who are the nurses who sort of link between intensive care and the normal wards. And she came and talked to me about possibly being moved on to a ward that day. And obviously that was all moving in the right direction and I desperately wanted that. But it was also a very scary prospect as well because there is, there's a security blanket you have in intensive care with having people there all the time because on the ward you don't have a nurse there all the time. And it was quite like passing a test. So she came sort of first thing in the morning at about eight and then I had to wait for the consultant to come round with his kind of army of doctors and students. And they all kind of huddled round my bed and kind of looked very serious at me and kind of looked at my notes and then sort of nodded at me and then went away, which somehow meant I was allowed to go down to the ward.

Interviewer: Yes. What was particularly good with the outreach?

> Well I just, I think they were very good at handholding almost, and they came and they were very efficient. There was a team of three of them and they started to come and see [me] in step down and then they came to see [me] every day until I had my trache out, which I think was about two weeks. So they would just monitor you and kind of, but they were very direct at talking to me and I felt, whereas the doctors generally didn't talk directly to me. They kind of talked to each other and would kind of shuffle on, whereas the nurses were very good at talking directly to me. And I think, and you could just see them working with other people as well. They were very efficient and it was sort of, they were there for when they needed to be there and then they weren't.

(http://www.healthtalkonline.org/Intensive_care/Intensive_care_Patients_experiences/
People/Interview/743/Category/70/Clip/6352/nurses#nurses)

Identifying the components of skilled nursing practice

WHAT THE REGULATORS SAY

The latest NMC (2010) competency framework provides the essential must-haves and must-dos that underpin practice through identifying the 'combination of skills, knowledge and attitudes, values and technical abilities that underpin safe and effective nursing practice and interventions' (p. 11). These competencies are organised into four domains:

1. professional values;
2. communication and interpersonal skills;
3. nursing practice and decision-making;
4. leadership, management and teamworking.

You can read about them in detail in the Appendix to this chapter.

In order to accomplish these competencies, the NMC (2010) has identified five accompanying essential skills clusters that students must achieve before registration as a nurse. These are:

- care, compassion and communication;
- organisational aspects of care;
- infection prevention and control;
- nutrition and fluid management;
- medicines management.

Each of these clusters has an associated set of key standards stating what the public can expect of the registered nurse (see the Professional Guidelines box) – you will be (or have been) working through your studies and practical work to achieve these.

WHAT SOME NURSING EDUCATORS SAY

Next, in order to continue to obtain a more contemporary view, I asked three nursing colleagues working in a variety of educational roles and settings what they thought were the essential skills required now for skilled professional practice (Box 3.7).

Drawing the threads for practice together – moving beyond the outline

The previous section in this chapter delineated the must-haves and must-dos of professional nursing practice – the competencies, skills, knowledge, attitudes and principles necessary for an outline of practice to be sketched so that you can successfully graduate as a safe, competent nurse. In that section, you saw the many lists of competencies tempered by just a few educators' comments that hint perhaps at something more to come – the richness of expert nursing; in reality, you will have experienced (or will be experiencing) this richness as the outlines of practice provided by the NMC are enriched by working with your teachers, mentors, role models and patients. The chapters in the second part of this book also capture that richness – the colour and depth of expert nursing – which you will aspire to as your career develops and better aligns with the ways through which patients and service users experience the totality of nursing.

This next section of the chapter lays out a conceptual framework of expert nursing practice that can be used to do two things: first, I will use it to draw together the threads for practice that have been put forward in the NMC (2010) standards and also in the RCN (2010) principles for nursing practice; second, you can use it as you read the chapters in Part Two of the book as a means of looking for expert practice and possibly critiquing it.

Many nurses have tried to reveal the expertise of nursing, but the most convincing work that I have found – and the one that resonates most with my own style of nursing –

KEY STANDARDS ASSOCIATED WITH THE FIVE ESSENTIAL SKILL CLUSTERS (NURSING AND MIDWIFERY COUNCIL, 2010)

Care, compassion and communication	Organisational aspects of care	Infection prevention and control	Nutrition and fluid management	Medicines management
As partners in the care process, people can trust a newly registered graduate nurse to provide collaborative care based on the highest standards, knowledge and competence.	People can trust the newly registered graduate nurse to treat them as partners and work with them to make a holistic and systematic assessment of their needs; to develop a personalised plan that is based on mutual understanding and respect for their individual situation promoting health and well-being, minimising risk of harm and promoting their safety at all times.	People can trust the newly registered graduate nurse to identify and take effective measures to prevent and control infection in accordance with local and national policy.	People can trust the newly registered graduate nurse to assist them to choose a diet that provides an adequate nutritional and fluid intake.	People can trust the newly registered graduate nurse to correctly and safely undertake medicines calculations.
People can trust the newly registered graduate nurse to engage in person centred care empowering people to make choices about how their needs are met when they are unable to meet them for themselves.	People can trust the newly registered graduate nurse to deliver nursing interventions and evaluate their effectiveness against the agreed assessment and care plan.	People can trust the newly registered graduate nurse to maintain effective standard infection control precautions and apply and adapt these to needs and limitations in all environments.	People can trust the newly registered graduate nurse to assess and monitor their nutritional status and in partnership, formulate an effective plan of care.	People can trust the newly registered graduate nurse to work within legal and ethical frameworks that underpin safe and effective medicines management.
People can trust the newly registered graduate nurse to respect them as individuals and strive to help them to preserve their dignity at all times.	People can trust the newly registered graduate nurse to safeguard children and adults from vulnerable situations and support and protect them from harm.	People can trust a newly registered graduate nurse to provide effective nursing interventions when someone has an infectious disease including the use of standard isolation techniques.	People can trust a newly registered graduate nurse to assess and monitor their fluid status and in partnership with them, formulate an effective plan of care.	People can trust the newly registered graduate nurse to work as part of a team to offer holistic care and a range of treatment options of which medicines may form a part.
People can trust a newly qualified graduate nurse to engage with them and their family or carers within their cultural environments in an acceptant and anti-discriminatory manner free from harassment and exploitation.	People can trust the newly registered graduate nurse to respond to their feedback and a wide range of other sources to learn, develop and improve services.	People can trust a newly registered graduate nurse to fully comply with hygiene, uniform and dress codes in order to limit, prevent and control infection.	People can trust the newly qualified graduate nurse to assist them in creating an environment that is conducive to eating and drinking.	People can trust the newly registered graduate nurse to ensure safe and effective practice in medicines management through comprehensive knowledge of medicines, their actions, risks and benefits.
			People can trust the newly qualified graduate nurse to ensure that those unable to take food by mouth receive adequate fluid and nutrition to meet their needs.	People can trust the newly registered graduate nurse to safely order, receive, store and dispose of medicines (including controlled drugs) in any setting.

People can trust the newly registered graduate nurse to engage with them in a warm, sensitive and compassionate manner.

People can trust the newly registered graduate nurse to engage therapeutically and actively listen to their needs and concerns, responding using skills that are helpful, providing information that is clear, accurate, meaningful and free from jargon.

People can trust the newly registered graduate nurse to protect and keep as confidential all information relating to them.

People can trust the newly registered graduate nurse to gain their consent based on sound understanding and informed choice prior to any intervention and that their rights in decision making and consent will be respected and upheld.

People can trust the newly registered graduate nurse to promote continuity when their care is to be transferred to another service or person.

People can trust the newly registered graduate nurse to be an autonomous and confident member of the multi-disciplinary or multi-agency team and to inspire confidence in others.

People can trust the newly registered graduate nurse to safely delegate to others and to respond appropriately when a task is delegated to them.

People can trust the newly registered graduate nurse to safely lead, co-ordinate and manage care.

People can trust the newly registered graduate nurse to work safely under pressure and maintain the safety of service users at all times.

People can trust a newly registered graduate nurse to enhance the safety of service users and identify and actively manage risk and uncertainty in relation to people, the environment, self and others.

People can trust the newly registered graduate nurse to work to prevent and resolve conflict and maintain a safe environment.

People can trust the newly registered graduate nurse to select and manage medical devices safely.

People can trust a newly registered graduate nurse to safely apply the principles of asepsis when performing invasive procedures and be competent in aseptic technique in a variety of settings.

People can trust the newly qualified nurse to act, in a variety of environments including the home care setting, to reduce risk when handling waste, including sharps, contaminated linen and when dealing with spillages of blood and other body fluids.

People can trust the newly registered graduate nurse to administer medicines safely and in a timely manner, including controlled drugs.

People can trust a newly registered graduate nurse to keep and maintain accurate records using information technology, where appropriate, within a multi-disciplinary framework as a leader and as part of a team and in a variety of care settings including at home.

People can trust a newly registered graduate nurse to work in partnership with people receiving medical treatments and their carers.

People can trust the newly registered graduate nurse to use and evaluate up-to-date information on medicines management and work within national and local policy guidelines.

People can trust the newly registered graduate nurse to demonstrate understanding and knowledge to supply and administer medicines via a patient group directive.

People can trust the newly registered graduate nurse to safely administer fluids when fluids cannot be taken independently.

Sue Green, Clinical Academic Career Senior Lecturer said:

Competence in delivering nutritional care of course [she is a specialist in nutrition]. Otherwise listening is a very underrated skill. A quiet presence. Relating the patient's concerns to other members of the team (with their permission of course). Competent and speedy undertaking of clinical skills. I would say my skills in really understanding the patient experience have developed as I have got older.

Mary Gobbi, Senior Lecturer in Nursing listed:

Ethics; communication; perseverance (from Nightingale); imagination (from Nightingale); patience; foresight; anticipation; reading signals and signs; ability to be a bricoleur; ability to look, and gaze; physiognomic perception.

She also gave examples from her research observations of nurses of silencing and mental intuition:

Silencing

P would stop and think ... moments of stillness, in the midst of the action. During this period she seemed to look around at the board [placement of patients], at bays and at the people. She would then make a decision. It also seemed important at this stage that she was not interrupted, as she was internally weighing the situation up. (Indeed if others were around her they would hold back and not interrupt, as if they were recognising the importance of the moment.) (P, month 6)

Mental intuition

The junior house officer asked for the [chest] drains to be removed. V didn't think that the drains should be removed. She described looking at the enrolled nurse 'we looked at one another', but neither acted. The consultant was subsequently 'cross' that the drains had been removed. V in discussing this said: 'I'll follow my instincts next time'. (V, month 3)

The former Prime Minister's Commission (Keen, 2010, p. 35) made us think about 'working with head, hands and heart to deliver high quality, compassionate care'. I wondered what this really meant until one of my colleagues used this to identify the key skills of an adult nurse.

Lisa Bayliss-Pratt, Regional Education Lead, wrote:

The key skills that adult nurses need from my point of view include:

Heart	*Compassion, advocacy, caring, listening, patience*
Hands	*Dexterity, conscientiousness, diligence*
Head	*Ability to make and take decisions, follow instructions and constructively challenge.*

comes from a group whose work originated in the UK (Rob Garbett, Sally Hardy, Kim Manley, Brendan McCormack and Angie Titchen). Their work, which crystallised when they worked together on the RCN Expertise in Practice Project (Box 3.8), has taken well over a decade to mature, and now presents a 'broad, interwoven vision of what is possible in nursing practice' (Manley et al., 2009, p. 3).

This vision is underpinned by two interlinked ideas: the first a conceptual framework of expert nursing practice, and the second an acknowledgement that the nurses practising within that framework need to create workplace environments that value person-centredness (person-centred systems), not only for the people receiving care, *but also* for the people providing it. Summarised in *Revealing Nursing Expertise Through Practitioner Inquiry* (Hardy et al., 2009), the conceptual framework has been strongly influenced not only by their own research studies, but also by the works of Patricia Benner and Tom Kitwood.

BOX 3.8 THE ROYAL COLLEGE OF NURSING (RCN) EXPERTISE IN PRACTICE PROJECT (MANLEY et al., 2005)

For 6 years between 1998 and 2004, the RCN undertook a project to better understand nursing practice expertise. The researchers undertaking the project focused on six cohorts of nurses working in a variety of clinical settings across the UK. The purpose of the project was to:

- recognise and value expertise in nursing practice;
- develop a recognition process for expertise in practice;
- develop further understanding of the concept of expertise within UK nursing and its different specialisms;
- explore the links between expertise and outcomes for service users and healthcare providers.

The research approach used in this project was a combination of emancipatory action research and fourth-generation evaluation. This involved 32 expert nurses (reduced by the end of the project to 22) working with a critical companion (approximately a facilitator) to explore and gather evidence of expertise through 360-degree reviews of their practice, observations of their practice and self-assessments reflecting on and in their practice in order to outline the elements of practice that the nurses thought classified them as being expert practitioners. These sources of evidence were then amalgamated into portfolios that were reviewed by a review panel.

Published as a report by the RCN and then later the subject of many papers, book chapters and books, the findings gave rise to the development of a conceptual framework for nursing expertise in the UK.

Nursing expertise (which, Manley et al. [2009] remind us, can take a career lifetime to develop) comprises five interdependent domains. The first domain – the domain of nursing practice expertise – focuses on 'achieving professional expertise and artistry in the nurse–patient relationship'. The remaining four domains focus on developing expertise in 'implementing and sustaining person-centred systems' through the 'facilitation of individuals, teams, systems, learning, research, inquiry, evaluation and change in practice so as to enable a culture of effectiveness to develop in the workplace' (Manley et al., 2009, p. 3).

The establishment of person-centred *systems* that go beyond any individual nurse's expertise ensures that care is delivered within cultures where the patient/service user experiences high-quality person-centred, evidence-based care from the team as a whole rather than just from an individual nurse – thus safeguarding the quality of that care. This culture of person-centredness also enables the development of expertise through learning from and enquiring about workplace experiences through either structured critical reflection or discussion, which in itself has the ability to alter practice (Manley et al., 2009; an idea supported also by Gobbi [2009], Gabbay and le May [2011] and other proponents of work-based learning).

Although the five domains of nursing expertise are now seen as interdependent, the domain of 'nursing practice expertise' was the first to emerge from the group's work with the RCN's Expertise in Practice Project and associated literature reviews and concept analyses.

This nursing practice expertise domain comprises eight attributes:

- Knowing the patient/client/colleague/organisation
- Holistic practical knowledge
- Saliency: knowing what matters and acting on it
- Moral integrity
- Skilled know-how
- Acting as a catalyst
- Creative, innovative and challenging behaviour
- Self-awareness.

The Professional Guidelines box provides more details of each of these attributes, as well as supporting references.

PROFESSIONAL GUIDELINES

THE ATTRIBUTES OF EXPERTISE (MANLEY et al., 2009, pp. 8–9)

Attributes (adapted from Manley et al., 2005)

Examples of empirical support in the literature since 1997

1. *Knowing the patient/client/colleague/organisation*
   Seeing patients as people who are unique, recognising and respecting their view of their illness or situation; getting to know the patient as person in the context of their own life to enable unique interventions and care that meet the needs of patients and their carers as they see them; recognising patients' patterns of behaviour and understanding how they are likely to react; forming rapport easily, being accessible on a person level and using one's own self to promote helping relationships; knowing when to relinquish control to patients/clients.

   Binnie and Titchen, 1999; Titchen, 2001; Titchen and McGinley, 2003; Bonner and Greenwood, 2006; McCormack and McCance, 2006

2. *Holistic practice knowledge*
   Integrating and using all kinds of knowledge in practice (e.g. theory, research, practical know-how, praxis, experiential, intuitive, aesthetic, personal); ongoing evaluation of, and learning from, new situations and embedding this knowledge for future use; using generic knowledge appropriately to individuals, groups, organisations and circumstances.

   Titchen, 2000; Titchen and McGinley, 2003; Donnelly, 2003; Judd, 2005; Kennedy, 2004; McCormack and McCance, 2006

3. *Saliency: knowing what matters and acting on it*
   Recognising intuitively and rationally what matters quickly and responding with immediate, seamless action; using skills appropriately and at the right time; listening and picking up verbal and non-verbal cues that can be missed by others; recognising patients', colleagues' and others' needs and reflecting these in action taken.

   Binnie and Titchen, 1999; Titchen, 2001 (skilled companionship); Taylor, 2002; Foley et al., 2002

4. *Moral integrity*

   Consciously promoting others' dignity and individuality and respecting their values and action without passing judgement; working and living one's values and beliefs without pushing them on others; providing information which enhances people's ability to solve problems and make decisions; being aware of one's own integrity and of setting the highest standards; aspiring to promote human flourishing for all involved in the clinical encounter through one's actions.

   Ersser, 1997; Binnie and Titchen, 1999; Titchen, 2000; Judd, 2005; Johnston and Smith, 2006; McCormack and McCance, 2006; McCormack and Titchen, 2006

5. *Skilled know-how*

   Adapting and responding skilfully and with consideration to each situation; enabling others through a willingness to share knowledge and skills, mobilising and using all available resources; seeing a path through a problem and inviting others on that journey.

   Binnie and Titchen, 1999; Titchen, 2001; Titchen and McGinley, 2003; Judd, 2005; Bonner and Greenwood, 2006

6. *Acting as a catalyst*

   Creating harmony and understanding, enabling new ways of working, and influencing colleagues' practice for better patient care, through education and role modelling.

   'Being a catalyst' describes the activities undertaken and considered necessary to keep the momentum of development continuing as well as the personal communication with individuals that enabled inclusivity.

   Binnie and Titchen, 1999; Titchen, 2001; Manley, 2001; Titchen and McGinley, 2003; Manley *et al.*, 2005

7. *Creative, innovative and challenging behaviour*

   Pursuing person-centred improvement relentlessly, being willing to take informed risks, that is, working ethically in a non-standard way, to achieve the best outcome for patients/clients; challenging practices and organisations to improve practices; encouraging others to develop a shared vision.

   Binnie and Titchen, 1999; Manley *et al.*, 2005; Bonner and Greenwood, 2006

8. *Self-awareness*

   Exploring and recognising one's own strengths and weaknesses; recognising one's scope of influence and impact; seeking self-improvement; articulating one's expertise and passion for nursing.

   Being self aware and attuned to others.

   Manley, 2001; Manley *et al.*, 2005; McCormack and McCance, 2006

Full details of these reference sources can be obtained at http://books.google.co.uk/ by searching for the Hardy et al. (2009) reference listed at the end of this chapter.

These attributes are associated with four factors required to enable the use of nurses' expertise: professional artistry, reflective ability, organisation of practice and autonomy and authority. Prominence is given to professional artistry since it:

enables the blending and melding of the [nursing practice expertise] attributes into unique configurations for each unique patient and context. The dimensions of professional artistry include, for example, different kinds of knowledge, ways of knowing, multiple intelligences [e.g. social, emotional, political], creative imagination and therapeutic use of self. (Manley et al., 2009, p. 10)

ENABLING FACTORS (MANLEY et al., 2009, pp. 7–8)

- *Professional artistry* – enables the individualising of care
- *Reflective ability* – reflexivity
- *Organisation of practice* – the capacity to critically control interactions in order to make an impact on the organisation by seeing the big picture
- *Autonomy and authority* – the capacity to make decisions and take responsibility, coupled with the willingness to challenge others if care is compromised

Valuing the person (whether a patient, client, family carer or professional carer) and their personhood ('a standing or status that is bestowed upon one human being, by others, in the context of relationship and social being. It implies recognition, respect and trust'; Kitwood, 1997, p. 8) is important not only in the way expertise is used in *patient care*, but also within the *organisational systems* that form the culture within which that care is being provided (Manley et al., 2009). Expert nurses therefore have both nursing practice expertise and expertise in creating and maintaining person-centred systems – in other words the culture of the ward/unit/clinic/practice/organisation within which care takes place. This expertise revolves around the four domains of (Manley et al., 2009, p. 12):

- facilitating learning and a work-based learning culture;
- facilitating inquiry, evaluation and evidence use;
- facilitating a culture of effectiveness through leadership;
- using consultancy approaches to foster self-sufficiency in problem-solving.

These domains are underpinned by numerous skills (Box 3.9), some of which we will return to in the next chapter.

Manley et al. (2009, pp. 22–3) draw clear links between levels of expertise in nursing practice and person-centred systems and a clinical career structure suggesting two parameters of expertise through which nurses weave their career progression. The first parameter focuses on 'A growing expertise and specialism with a specific client group' (e.g. nurse practitioners in general medical practice, emergency nurse practitioners in minor injuries units or clinical nurse specialists working with particular groups of patients with acute or long-term conditions). These practitioners, they suggest, are associated primarily with the delivery of client-centred care.

The second parameter focuses on 'A growing expertise in the domains necessary to develop person-centred systems'. This group of practitioners will include, for example, team or clinical leaders, managers with roles that link practice and management, practice development nurses, lecturer practitioners and consultant nurses. They will all, to a greater or lesser extent, have to share their time between giving care directly and creating an environment within which patient-centred, evidence-based, high-quality care is provided. A good example of this parameter is the consultant nurse who uses expertise in nursing practice combined with expertise in the development of workplace cultures to facilitate the delivery of high-quality care throughout the patient's journey, regardless of who is giving that care, where that care is given and when. Nursing practice career frameworks, therefore, need to be underpinned by a 'spectrum of expertise' (p. 4), which develops over time, spanning the domains focused on the nurse–patient relationship *and* the system of care delivery.

To conclude, expert nurses, if we use Manley et al.'s (2009) conceptual framework, have highly specialised practice-focused skills, which are amplified by the more generalist skills associated with maintaining person-centred systems. Both sets of skills are needed in order to deliver high-quality care by the nursing team to patients, service users and their carers: these will be examined in more detail as this book progresses.

Further information

You might find it interesting to read more about the importance of seeing the person behind the patient in the following two texts:

- Point of Care (2009) *Are You Seeing the Person in the Patient?* London: King's Fund
- Brendan McCormack and Tanya McCance (2010) *Person-centred Nursing*. Oxford: Wiley-Blackwell.

Patricia Benner's (1984) classic text *From Novice to Expert: Excellence and power in clinical nursing practice* (Addison-Wesley, Menlo Park, California) is a book that you should not miss if you want to see how her research sheds light on nurses' journeys towards expertise.

In addition, the Foundation of Nursing Studies (FoNS) has launched a new website – www.fons.org – the first of its kind, to help nurses lead innovation and change in order to ensure the delivery of care that is high quality and evidence-based, and meets patients' needs. Through it, the Centre for Nursing Innovation provides access to an online community where healthcare practitioners can discuss issues and share expertise. There is also a library of useful reports and case studies, tools and resources that can be used in the workplace and for access to practice development programmes and funding.

Appendix

THE NMC COMPETENCY FRAMEWORK SUMMARISED

The first domain – professional values – reminds nurses (Nursing and Midwifery Council, 2010) that they:

> must act first and foremost to care for and safeguard the public. They must practise autonomously and be responsible and accountable for safe, compassionate, person-centred, evidence-based nursing that respects and maintains dignity and human rights. They must show professionalism and integrity and work within recognised professional, ethical and legal frameworks. They must work in partnership with other health and social care professionals and agencies, service users, their carers and families in all settings, including the community, ensuring that decisions about care are shared.

(All quotes in the Appendix are taken from pp. 13–21 of Nursing and Midwifery Council, 2010.)

The Professional Guidelines box provides a summary of the detailed competencies.

PROFESSIONAL GUIDELINES

PROFESSIONAL VALUES (NURSING AND MIDWIFERY COUNCIL, 2010)
The detailed competencies for this domain place emphasis on holistic, non-judgemental, caring and sensitive practice that:
- is inclusive challenging inequality, discrimination and exclusion accessing care
- supports and promotes the health, wellbeing, rights and dignity of people, groups, communities and populations
- creates partnerships with service users, carers, families, groups, communities and organisations
- recognises and manages risk.

In order to do this successfully nurses need to

- understand their various roles, responsibilities and functions: appropriately use these to meet the changing needs of people, groups, communities and populations
- work collaboratively with other health and social care professionals
- be responsible and accountable for keeping their knowledge and skills up-to-date
- improve performance and the safety and quality of care through evaluation, supervision and appraisal
- recognise their limits and seek advice from others as needed
- appreciate the value of evidence in practice, be able to understand, appraise and apply research and relevant theory and identify areas for further investigation.

The second domain – communication and interpersonal skills – reminds nurses that they:

> must use excellent communication and interpersonal skills. Their communications must always be safe, effective, compassionate and respectful. They must communicate effectively using a wide range of strategies and interventions including the effective use of communication technologies. Where people have a disability, nurses must be able to work with service users and others to obtain the information needed to make reasonable adjustments that promote optimum health and enable equal access to services. …

Adult nurses must demonstrate the ability to listen with empathy. They must be able to respond warmly and positively to people of all ages who may be anxious, distressed, or facing problems with their health and well-being. The detailed competencies for communication and interpersonal skills are also shown in a Professional Guidelines box here.

PROFESSIONAL GUIDELINES

COMMUNICATION AND INTERPERSONAL SKILLS (NURSING AND MIDWIFERY COUNCIL, 2010)

The detailed competencies for this domain emphasise the importance of:

- building partnerships and therapeutic relationships through safe, effective and non-discriminatory communication taking account of individual differences, capabilities and needs
- using a range of communication skills and technologies to support person-centred care enabling informed choice and shared decision making whilst enhancing quality and safety
- using the full range of communication methods – verbal, non-verbal and written, to acquire, interpret and record knowledge and understanding of people's needs
- being aware of your own values and beliefs and their impact on communication
- promoting self-care with people with acute and long-term conditions
- recognising when people are anxious or distressed and responding therapeutically and effectively to promote their wellbeing, manage personal safety and resolve conflict

- knowing when to consult others and how to make referrals for advocacy, mediation or arbitration
- using therapeutic principles to engage, maintain and, where appropriate, disengage from professional caring relationships, and respecting professional boundaries
- encouraging health-promoting behaviour through education, role modelling and effective communication
- maintaining accurate, clear and complete records, including the use of electronic formats, using appropriate and plain language
- respecting individual rights to confidentiality and keeping information secure and confidential in accordance with the law and relevant ethical, regulatory and local frameworks
- sharing personal information with others when the interests of safety and protection override the need for confidentiality.

The third domain (also summarised in a Professional Guidelines box) focuses on nursing practice and decision-making, emphasising that all nurses should:

> practise autonomously, compassionately, skillfully and safely, and must maintain dignity and promote health and wellbeing. They must assess and meet the full range of essential physical and mental health needs of people of all ages who come into their care. Where necessary they must be able to provide safe and effective immediate care to all people prior to accessing or referring to specialist services irrespective of their field of practice. All nurses must also meet more complex and coexisting needs for people in their own nursing field of practice, in any setting including hospital, community and at home. All practice should be informed by the best available evidence and comply with local and national guidelines. Decision-making must be shared with service users, carers and families and informed by critical analysis of a full range of possible interventions, including the use of up-to-date technology. All nurses must also understand how behaviour, culture, socioeconomic and other factors, in the care environment and its location, can affect health, illness, health outcomes and public health priorities and take this into account in planning and delivering care.

PROFESSIONAL GUIDELINES

NURSING PRACTICE AND DECISION-MAKING (NURSING AND MIDWIFERY COUNCIL, 2010)

The detailed competencies for this domain emphasise the importance of:

- using up-to-date knowledge and evidence to assess, plan, deliver and evaluate care, communicate findings, influence change, promote health and best practice
- carrying out comprehensive, systematic nursing assessments taking account of relevant physical, social, cultural, psychological, spiritual, genetic, environmental factors, in partnership with service users and others

- making person-centred, evidence-based judgments and decisions, in partnership with others involved in the care process, to ensure high quality care
- recognising when clinical decisions require others' specialist knowledge and expertise and consulting/referring accordingly
- applying relevant knowledge from the life, behavioural and social sciences to health, ill health, disability, ageing and death
- ascertaining and responding to the physical/social/psychological needs of people, groups and communities
- providing safe, competent, person-centred care in partnership with service users, paying special attention to changing health needs during different life stages, including progressive illness and death, loss and bereavement
- understanding public health principles, priorities and practice in order to recognise and respond to the major causes and social determinants of health, illness and inequalities
- practising safely by being aware of the correct use, limitations and hazards of common interventions, including nursing activities, treatments, and the use of medical devices and equipment: evaluating their use, appropriately reporting any concerns and modifying care
- contributing to the collection of local and national data and the formulation of policy on risks, hazards and adverse outcomes
- recognising and interpreting signs of normal and deteriorating mental and physical health and promptly responding to maintain or improve the health and comfort of the service user, acting to keep them and others safe
- optimising health and wellbeing through educational support, facilitation and therapeutic nursing interventions
- promoting self-care and management when possible, helping people to make choices, involving families and carers where appropriate
- recognising and acting when a person is at risk and needs extra support and protection
- evaluating care to improve clinical decision-making, quality and outcomes, amending the plan of care, where necessary, and communicating changes to others.

Leadership, management and teamworking comprise the fourth domain, which emphasises that:

> all nurses must be professionally accountable and use clinical governance processes to maintain and improve nursing practice and standards of healthcare. They must be able to respond autonomously and confidently to planned and uncertain situations, managing themselves and others effectively. They must create and maximise opportunities to improve services. They must also demonstrate the potential to develop further management and leadership skills during their period of preceptorship and beyond.

Adult nurses in particular:

must be able to provide leadership in managing adult nursing care, understand and coordinate interprofessional care when needed, and liaise with specialist teams. They must be adaptable and flexible, and able to take the lead in responding to the needs of people of all ages in a variety of circumstances, including situations where immediate or urgent care is needed. They must recognise their leadership role in disaster management, major incidents and public health emergencies, and respond appropriately according to their levels of competence.

A summary of the detailed competencies here is given in the Professional Guidelines box below.

PROFESSIONAL GUIDELINES

LEADERSHIP, MANAGEMENT AND TEAMWORKING (NURSING AND MIDWIFERY COUNCIL, 2010)

The detailed competencies for this domain emphasise the importance of:

- acting as change agents and providing leadership through quality improvement and service development to enhance people's wellbeing and experiences of healthcare
- systematically evaluating care and using those findings to help improve people's experience and care outcomes and to shape future services
- identifying priorities and managing time and resources effectively in order to maintain or enhance the quality of care
- being self-aware and recognising how your own values, principles and assumptions may affect practice
- maintaining your own personal and professional development, learning from experience, through supervision, feedback, reflection and evaluation
- facilitating nursing students and others to develop their competence, using a range of professional and personal development skills
- working independently as well as in teams
- taking the lead in coordinating, delegating and supervising care safely, managing risk and remaining accountable for the care given
- working effectively across professional and agency boundaries, actively involving and respecting others' contributions to integrated person-centred care
- knowing when, and how, to communicate with and refer to other professionals and agencies in order to respect the choices of service users and others
- promoting shared decision making, to deliver positive outcomes and to coordinate smooth, effective transition within and between services and agencies.

References

Committee on Nursing (1972) *Report of the Committee on Nursing* (the Briggs Report). London: HMSO.

Department of Health (2010) *Equity and Excellence: Liberating the NHS*. London: Department of Health.

Gabbay J , le May A (2011) *Practice Based Evidence for Healthcare: Clinical mindlines*. London: Routledge.

Gobbi M (2009) Learning nursing in a workplace community: the generation of professional capital. In: *Communities of Practice in Health and Social Care*, le May A (ed.). Oxford: Wiley-Blackwell, pp. 66–82.

Hardy S, Titchen A, McCormack B, Manley K (eds) (2009) *Revealing Nursing Expertise Through Practitioner Inquiry*. Oxford: Wiley-Blackwell.

Keen A (2010) Front Line Care: Report by the Prime Minister's Commission on the Future of Nursing and Midwifery in England. Retrieved from: http://cnm.independent.gov.uk (accessed 2 January 2011).

Kitwood T (1997) On being a person. In: *Dementia Reconsidered: The person comes first*, Kitwood T (ed.). Milton Keynes: Open University Press.

Manley K, Hardy S, Titchen A, Garbett R, McCormack B (2005) *Changing Patients' Worlds Through Nursing Practice Expertise. A Royal College of Nursing Research Report 1998–2004*. London: RCN Institute.

Manley K, Titchen A, Hardy S (2009) From artistry in practice to expertise in developing person-centred systems: a clinical career framework. In: *Revealing Nursing Expertise Through Practitioner Inquiry*, Hardy S, Titchen A, McCormack B, Manley K (eds). Oxford: Wiley-Blackwell, pp. 3–30.

Maslin A (1999) *Nursing the World: Celebrating the past, claiming the future*. London: NT Books.

Nursing and Midwifery Council (2008) *The Code: Standards of conduct, performance and ethics for nurses and midwives*. London: NMC.

Nursing and Midwifery Council (2010) *Standard for Pre-registration Nursing Education*. London: NMC.

Royal College of Nursing (2003) Defining Nursing. Retrieved from: http://www.rcn.org.uk/__data/assets/pdf_file/0003/78564/001983.pdf (accessed 27 May 2011).

Royal College of Nursing (2010) Principles of Nursing Practice. Retrieved from: http://www.rcn.org.uk/development/practice/principles (accessed 27 May 2011).

Turner P (2007) Caring for the 'whole person': spiritual aspects of care. In: *Principles of Professional Studies in Nursing*, Brown J, Libberton P (eds). Basingstoke: Palgrave Macmillan, pp. 96–110.

Chapter 4

DEVELOPING EXPERT PRACTICE

Andrée le May

LEARNING OUTCOMES

You will learn the following from this chapter:

- **How leadership, research utilisation and the development of oneself and others are essential for the creation and delivery of expert practice**
- **How practice is developed through not only the use of the best evidence in decision-making, but also experience in creatively implementing that evidence**
- **How nursing has developed outside the boundaries of traditional healthcare providers to businesses in the private sector**
- **How skills of entrepreneurship are essential to the development of modern nursing**

OVERVIEW

When Dave Barton and I were designing the structure of this textbook, we started by thinking about the key elements of high-quality nursing practice, and a number of interlinked themes emerged, the key ones being the use of safe clinical skills, leadership, research utilisation and the ongoing development of oneself and others; these themes run throughout this book and are pivotal to the growth of expert, high-quality practice. In Chapter 3, they featured as core elements of professional practice in the Nursing and Midwifery Council (NMC) standards, the Royal College of Nursing (RCN) principles and Manley et al.'s conceptual framework of expertise. The creation of what Manley et al. (2009) describe as person-centred systems (or cultures) is underpinned by three of these themes – leadership, research utilisation, and personal development and the development of others; the purpose of this chapter is to discover more about these. Although each is explored in separate sections, they are in reality intricately linked and hard to prise apart.

About the author

You can read Andrée's story of her nursing career on p. 49.

Leadership – bringing about a culture of effectiveness

This section starts with a poem by Sue Duke. Sue is a clinical leader working as a consultant practitioner and senior lecturer in cancer and palliative care at the University of Southampton. She wrote her leadership synthesis poem as part of her exploration of consultant practice for her PhD. This poem illustrates how clinical leaders bring together and shape the substance of their leadership in order to develop a distinctive leadership style grounded in and relevant to their practice. This style is influenced by who they are, the skills that they possess, the people who have influenced them, the people with whom they work, the organisation within which they work and the work that has to be done. All of these are clearly visible, to me, in Sue's poem. The poem shows how leadership goes far beyond the theory presented in textbooks and can become an integral part of an expert practitioner's practice requiring her or him to be in tune with not only others and their surroundings, but also themselves.

AN INSIGHT INTO LEADERSHIP

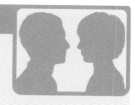

I know leadership by how I be, not by how I do, my theory-in-action: knowing-in-being.

Theoretical concepts like vision collaboration, facilitation, inadequately capture the essence of my leadership experience. I know leadership by a gentleness, stillness within me, by space in my being creating embodied meaning, spiritual knowing of relationships.

When I act from this knowing-in-being

I lead. My practice congruent with my beliefs and values, practice constructed through relationships.

Co-relationships co-creating the rhythm and tempo, pitch and harmony, of nursing practice.

At the best of times, when nursing practice is in tune within these relationships, leadership is fluid.

Knowing-in-being joyful, effortless. Leadership enriched by mutual, shared, skilled-understanding.

At the worst of times, when nursing practice provokes discordance in relationships, leadership is stilted.

Knowing-in-being painful, effort-full. Leadership thwarted by competing thoughts, rival emotions.

At these times the space within me is filled to capacity.

My being like a jumble sale, messy, cluttered, higgledy-piggledy. Knowledge of how to respond camouflaged amongst the jumble. Most-times I catch a glimmer

of how to respond. Out of the corner of my eye see the jumble sale treasure: tacitly perceive how to be, to lead; act from within me.

To catch a glimmer of how to respond requires me to trust my self, my practice.

My trust in my self sometimes challenged by pre-written scripts deep within me. When nurse-doctor relation scripts are enacted, knowing-in-being is tension between

obeying the rules:
following the script
by playing my part;
or re-writing the script:
to portray my part.

A tension between
holding my tongue so
that I do not say what I
    really think,
express my frustration at
    outdated
assumptions about
nurses' place in
relationships;
and holding my voice,
so that I am heard.

Whilst I describe my
knowing-in-being
as consequently
paralysed, thwarted,
holding my voice, as
in voicing my voice,
is an active act,
models my values:
respecting colleagues
and their point of view
whilst advocating
patients' needs, choices.

Whilst my voice might
    not
be in harmony,
indeed discordant,
it is not silent.

My trust in my self
is sometimes challenged
by expectations
and workload demands.

My self transformed from
being, to doing
what's needed to get
through the day. No room
for relationships –
morally valued
still – just exhausted
by unrelenting
patient distress, by
lack of resources.

Just exhausted by
the exploding health
care changes, by
lack of personal
leadership support.

Knowing-in-being
transformed to doing,
working from without.

In the middle
of the best and worst
    times,
are every-day-times
when I respond by
acting from within;
knowing-in-being
congruent self-trust.

Fashioned by tensions,
these everyday times

are characterised
by decisions through
potential choices.

Demonstrating how
people facing death
and bereavement can
be well cared for, their
choices respected.

Demonstrating how
resources foster
good care, lobbying
acquisition and
fair distribution.

Demonstrating how
making and sustaining
lateral networks
build capacity,
foster shared learning.

Demonstrating my
nursing knowledge by
substantiating
clinical decisions,
showing my thinking.

Making my research
knowledge explicit,
being respectful
of others' knowing,
whilst offering mine.

Working with meanings
to sensitise care
contextually

and managing the
chaos that results.

Managing the pull
within hybridity.
Two identities,
yet neither a place
in which to belong.

Nurse consultancy
embodies the quest
for clinical nurse
leadership. My lived
experience not
always congruent
with the rhetoric.

I know leadership
by how I be, my
knowing-in-being
constantly weathered
by instrumental
challenges, sub-scripts,
contradictory
expectations, lack
of time, of staff, of
leadership support.

If I can hold voice
in the midst of these
elements, I lead.

If I can hold true,
to relationships,
then I lead with grace.

Poem copyright Sue Duke

Leadership is a multifaceted phenomenon that can be displayed through a myriad of often quite personal styles. Consider for a moment, before we delve into some theoretical aspects of leadership, your own style of leadership (see the Activity box).

THINKING ABOUT LEADERSHIP: WHAT SORT OF LEADERSHIP STYLE DO YOU HAVE?

Think of an example of when you were the leader. It could have been when you were leading a team of people in order to achieve a task (regardless of size or difficulty) or leading on decisions about the care of a patient/service user. It could have been when you were a senior student or when you were qualified. How would you describe your leadership style? What were the key characteristics of it? Think about the people you were leading. Try to find one or two of them and ask them to describe your leadership style. Would your description match theirs? If not, why not?

Jot down and keep your answers so that you can think about them again after you've read Table 4.1 on leadership styles.

Nurses lead in many ways and in many situations. They lead projects, teams, groups of students through mentorship, organisations and episodes of care – and whatever it is that they are leading requires strong and effective leadership in order to successfully create and sustain a culture of effectiveness. Leadership is essentially about our relationships with other people and the way we constructively influence them to deliver effective care.

A DEFINITION OF LEADERSHIP

Leadership involves influence, it occurs among people, those people intentionally desire significant changes, and the changes reflect purposes shared by leaders and followers. *Influence* means that the relationship between people is not passive; however, also inherent in this definition is the concept that influence is multidirectional and non-coercive.

(Daft, 1999, p. 5)

Leaders often achieve influence by adopting a particular style of leadership. The three most commonly described styles of leadership are authoritarian, democratic and laissez-faire (Table 4.1): each is different and depends largely on what the leader is focusing on – be that organising work or scheduling work activities; or defining roles and responsibilities; or building camaraderie, respect, trust and liking between the leader and his/her followers. (Read more about how these styles of leadership might impact on nursing staff in Cox and le May, 2007.)

Some styles will of course work better than others: although this is primarily associated with the leader's abilities, skills and personal qualities (Box 4.1) the success (or not) of a leadership style is also intricately linked to the situation within which the leadership happens.

Each situation is a distinctive, rather complex occurrence for which many things need to be taken into account, for example what the task is that has to be achieved, how well formulated the task is, what the leader's relationship is to the people she or he is leading (followers) towards achieving that task, and the extent to which followers can or cannot

Table 4.1 Styles of leadership (reproduced with permission from Cox and le May, 2007, p. 160 based on Mullins, 1999)

	Authoritarian style	Democratic style	Laissez-faire style
Primary focus	The work to be done. Completing the task to a high standard	Development of individuals and the team. Delegation used as a means to develop others	Enabling others to manage and control their own work
Focus of power	Maintaining power and control over the work	The team	Individual members of the team
Normal behaviour	The leader Initiating structure by defining roles and responsibilities for all team members. Planning the work to be undertaken each day. Making decisions and expecting others to follow the directions given	Sharing leadership functions among the team. Acting as part of the team Seeking opinions of staff in the decision-making process. Interacting with all members of the group	Allowing individuals to work autonomously and only assisting individuals when required Allowing individuals to work autonomously and only assisting individuals when required
Leaders' expectations of others	Feedback from staff on progress of work. Refer/check decisions with the leader	Take on responsibility and develop skills	Work autonomously. Request assistance when required

BOX 4.1   LEADERSHIP ABILITIES, SKILLS AND PERSONAL QUALITIES

LEADERSHIP ABILITIES AND SKILLS
Embodying values
Articulation of vision
Creativity and innovation
Responsiveness and flexibility
Decision-making and taking
Motivating self
Motivating others
Releasing talent
Judging success
Telling others
(London Regional Office, 2000)

Required for setting direction
Political astuteness
Drive for results
Broad scanning
Intellectual flexibility
Seizing the future

Required for delivering the service
Collaborative working
Effective and strategic influencing
Empowering others
Holding to account
Leading change through people
(NHS Leadership Centre, 2002)

PERSONAL QUALITIES
Enthusiasm
Integrity
Courage
Humility
(Daft, 1999)

Self-belief
Self-awareness
Self-management
Drive for improvement
Personal integrity
(NHS Leadership Centre, 2002)

Integrity
Enthusiasm
Warmth
Calmness
Being tough but fair
'Possessing and exemplifying the qualities expected or required in' the group of people that they are working with. Most importantly perhaps 'it's the juxtaposition of qualities – the patterns of qualities – that matters most.'
(Adair, 2010, pp. 8–10)

trust and respect the leader. The most effective leaders take all of this into consideration and select the most appropriate style for each situation.

Hersey and Blanchard (1977) were the first, in their theory of situational leadership, to emphasise the need for leaders to be adaptable. They proposed that leaders, in order to be effective, needed to pay particular attention to the maturity, ability and motivation of the team or individuals they were leading, and to adapt their style accordingly. Four leadership styles were identified depending on the extent to which followers needed to be directed to achieve the goal or just supported in doing this:

- directing: the leader decides what to do;
- coaching: the leader works alongside and talks to followers, but it is still the leader who decides what to do;
- supporting: the leader works with the followers and together they decide what is required;
- delegating: the leader allows the followers to decide what to do.

In order to work like this, the leader needs to be able to determine which leadership style to adopt. Hersey and Blanchard offered some pointers about this, suggesting that if followers are very motivated and competent, a delegating leader will work, but if they are the opposite – poorly motivated and lacking competence – a directing leader is required. If followers lack motivation but are highly competent, a supporting style may be appropriate, whereas if they are highly motivated but have little competence in relation to the task, a coaching style will be required. Their theory is often presented pictorially (Fig. 4.1).

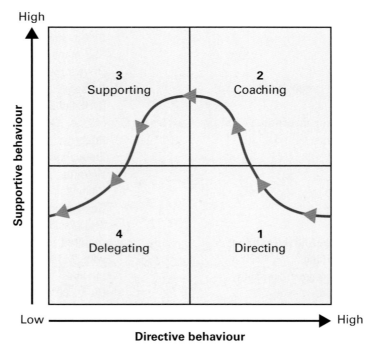

Figure 4.1 Situational leadership (reproduced from http://ollhoff.com/writings/leadership/classic_models.htm)

Although the emphasis on adaptability in Hersey and Blanchard's theory makes good sense, it seems to have lost sight of the often complex interrelationship between the team, its members, the task and the context within which leadership is happening. It is important also to remember that, in some situations, people you might expect to be leaders will not be the right leaders at all – in this instance, they will become followers; this is usually associated with the knowledge that they possess and its appropriateness, or otherwise, to a given situation (Adair, 2010).

Adair's (2010) action-centred leadership theory moves closer to recognising the interconnectedness and complex interplay between the leader, the nature of the task to be achieved, the needs of the team of people involved in achieving the task and the needs of the individuals in that team. Often depicted as three overlapping circles (Fig. 4.2), the essential components of his model are:

- the need to achieve the task;
- the need to maintain the team's cohesiveness;
- the needs of the individuals involved as people.

Successful leadership is about what leaders do (action) to ensure that *all* of these needs are met. To lose sight of any one of the circles means jeopardising the remaining ones.

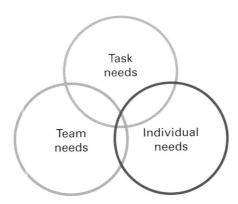

Figure 4.2 Action-centred leadership (reproduced from http://kairology.com/wp-content/uploads/2009/02/picture-1.png)

Adair (2010) gives us some hints about what a leader should *do* (key functions) in order to achieve the task and hold the team together. The functions revolve around organising and planning:

- setting objectives to show a clear purpose;
- planning for achieving the objectives and agreeing that plan;
- briefing everyone involved so they know the objectives and the plan;
- controlling, supervising and monitoring (keeping the work of the group on track);
- evaluating so that the team and individuals can obtain effective feedback.

The skill in leadership lies in knowing which function to pay attention to when and then how to do that well with the people you are working with – this last bit being perhaps where different leaders will bring in their different personal qualities and styles.

Handy's (1993, p. 103) 'best-fit approach' also addresses the need for leaders to be adaptable and to take into account the four influencing factors: themselves (the leader), their followers, the task and the environment of the organisation within which the leaders and followers have to achieve the task – the context.

All of these approaches emphasise a directive yet adaptive way to lead people. Recently, however, there has been a movement away from this style of leading, with leadership approaches focusing more and more on inspiring people to change rather than on directing them. Some ways to inspire others to change are best summed up by Kouzes and Posner (2002) (Box 4.2).

BOX 4.2   HOW TO INSPIRE OTHERS

Being able to inspire others requires leaders to do the following.

Model the way
'Modeling means going first, living the behaviors you want others to adopt. This is leading from the front. People will believe not what they hear leaders say but what they see leaders consistently do. People may believe the leader in preference to the plan.'

Inspire a shared vision
'People are motivated most not by fear or reward, but by ideas that capture their imagination. Note that this is not so much about having a vision, but communicating it so effectively that others take it as their own.'

Challenge the process
'Leaders thrive on and learn from adversity and difficult situations. They are early adopters of innovation.'

Enable others to act
'Encouragement and exhortation is not enough. People must feel able to act and then must have the ability to put their ideas into action and work collaboratively.'

Encourage the heart
'People act best of all when they are passionate about what they are doing. Leaders unleash the enthusiasm of their followers often with stories and passions of their own. People like to know that their efforts have been appreciated.'

Kouzes and Posner, 2002

Sometimes, when the change that is desired will have a major impact across an organisation, this type of inspirational leadership is referred to as being transformational. For well over a decade, NHS policy and practice has aspired to this kind of leadership, believing that it is the ability to rapidly transform services and organisations. However, there is a growing recognition that reliance on transformational leadership may have been somewhat idealistic as, despite very committed marketing by politicians and policy makers, it has not achieved the anticipated step-change in service development or delivery.

Regardless of individual style, there are, when we think about leading in nursing practice, some key elements that we need to keep at the centre of that process if we are to deliver effective care and to create and sustain the more person-centred cultures that were mentioned in Chapter 3. These key elements include:

- first, the importance of focusing on the task, the team, the individual and the context within which the leadership is happening;
- second, the importance of having the right knowledge for the situation and, as a consequence, being respected and trusted by the team for that;
- third, acknowledging that the sort of leadership that is required in everyday practice is rarely only that which has become known as transformational, and that leadership-for-practice may instead be better aligned with Binney et al.'s (2005) ideas on living leadership – being realistic, connecting with others and asking for help when it is needed. The characteristics of living leadership are summarised in Box 4.3, and a presentation is available for viewing at http://www.ashridge.org.uk/website/content.nsf/wCON/ Living+Leadership?opendocument
- fourth, acknowledging that the centrality of the patient must never be forgotten and should constantly remain uppermost in our minds. The patient-centredness of practice needs to guide our actions, as McNichol and Hamer's (2006) three-dimensional model of health systems leadership and management demonstrates. This model shows how, in order to achieve purposeful leadership and management, the leader needs to consider three interrelated and interdependent points – patient-centred care, effective teams and understanding oneself – all of which are affected by (and will in turn affect) the context within which care happens.

BOX 4.3 LIVING LEADERSHIP – THE KEY FEATURES

Leadership happens between people: it is the product of the interactions between leaders, followers and the context within which they are working.

Ordinary acts of everyday leadership include: speaking your truth, tackling uncomfortable issues, connecting people and organisations, and confronting people who are not performing.

Leaders face particular pressures: these include high expectations, constantly changing environments, anxiety and the requirement to convert sometimes unrealistic visions into realistic outcomes, and the need for a clear lead from above that may never come.

The art of the possible is important – being too idealistic can end in frustration and failure. Transformations often ended up with endings different from those that were planned.

Effective leaders use themselves with skill. They are not perfect. They realise that they will make progress only if they can release and harness the skills and intelligence of others.

Binney et al., 2005

Good leadership enables the creation of confidence, trust and respect among people, within teams, and between patients, their relatives and their nurses. Good leadership enables people to thrive, to be inspired, to take advantage of professional development opportunities and to grow themselves into good leaders or good followers. Good leadership enables the delivery of high-quality care within environments where people are valued. Good leadership is the bedrock of excellence in nursing.

Research utilisation

Since the 1970s, increasing prominence has been given to the use of research findings, from a variety of research designs, to ensure that clinically effective nursing and a high quality of care is delivered to patients by all members of the nursing team. In order to provide the best care, every nurse (qualified or student) needs to make every effort to use, as Cullum et al. (2008, p. 2) put it, 'valid, relevant research-based information in [their] decision making'.

Although this sounds easy, it is in fact a rather complex undertaking that requires you to find, often through searching the literature, the right research to suit your clinical needs, and then to determine whether that research is good enough to use (rigorous) and also clinically relevant to the person or group of people you want to use it with. If it is, then you have to convince other people – colleagues and patients – to change what they usually do in order to incorporate the research into their practice. You will have to draw on your leadership and change management skills to do this successfully. Once this change has been achieved, an evaluation of the success, or otherwise, of the research-based care needs to be made and fed back to anyone who is interested and/or needs to know.

Any or all of these steps may be further complicated by a process whereby the research-based information has to compete with other sorts of information before it is implemented into practice (Gabbay and le May, 2011; le May, 2009a; Rycroft-Malone et al., 2004). These competing sources of information stem from several areas: clinical experience – your own and or others'; patient/client/carer experience; central or local policies/guidelines; and information from the local context (e.g. the research might conflict with local policy or there may be insufficient resources or skilled personnel to implement it) (le May, 1999; Rycroft-Malone et al., 2004).

If the research findings are suitable for implementation, another set of challenges presents itself – those primarily associated with people's attitudes towards research and change and the resources available (Box 4.4). The effects of these barriers are often ameliorated by a series of opportunities (Box 4.5) and by involving skilled change agents, opinion leaders or champions (see the Activity box on finding more out about research and change management) in the process of implementation if research utilisation is to go beyond an individual nurse providing research-based care to an individual patient.

BOX 4.4 PRACTITIONERS' PERCEIVED BARRIERS TO RESEARCH-BASED PRACTICE

Attitudes
- Lack of cooperation
- Lack of motivation
- Fear
- Resistance to change
- Acceptance of ritualised or traditional practice

Beliefs
- Research will not make a difference
- Research data are not appropriate
- Conviction that current practice is OK

Professional relationships
- Medical staff block implementation
- Medical staff consider nursing research to be substandard
- Nursing colleagues are uncooperative

- Senior staff are resistant to change
- Low grading of research staff and often insecure posts

Organisational issues
- Time
- Pressure of workload
- Too much change

Educational issues
- Practitioners unaware of or unable to access research
- Lack of skills in critical appraisal
- Lack of skills in change management
- Research reports are jargonistic
- Implementing new research may mean developing different clinical skills

Adapted and updated from Le May et al., 1998

BOX 4.5 OPPORTUNITIES TO DEVELOP RESEARCH-BASED PRACTICE

Organisational support
- Specific research and development strategy for health trust or for nursing
- Enhanced links with education providers
- Funding for courses and workshops; clinical academic career structures
- Specific appointments with an emphasis on research and practice/teaching
- Identification and support of champions for nursing

New 'structures'
- Research fora
- Research awareness groups
- Proactive research/ethics committees
- Research centres
- Nursing development units

- Collaborations for Leadership in Applied Health Research and Care (CLAHRC) funded by National Institute for Health Research (NIHR) at the Department of Health

Interprofessional relationships
- Multiprofessional initiatives, e.g. guideline development
- Multidisciplinary research: multiagency research

Changing individuals
- Greater uptake of continuing education
- Recognition of the importance of research by individuals
- Diploma and degree courses increasing individual skills and knowledge

Adapted and updated from Le May et al., 1998

Some researchers, practitioners and academics have formulated frameworks which, if followed, might improve the utilisation of research in practice. The best known of these are summarised in Box 4.6. Further details of these and several other models and frameworks for implementing evidence-based practice can be found in a comprehensive textbook edited by Rycroft-Malone and Bucknall (2010).

BOX 4.6   FRAMEWORKS FOR IMPLEMENTING RESEARCH IN PRACTICE

PROMOTING ACTION ON RESEARCH IMPLEMENTATION IN HEALTH SERVICES (PARIHS) FRAMEWORK (RYCROFT-MALONE, 2010)

This framework emphasises that the success of implementation depends on the relationship between key factors:
- the nature of the evidence (whether it is research, clinical experience or patient experience)
- the context within which it is implemented (this includes the culture of the organisation, leadership and the potential for evaluation)
- this implementation is facilitated (this depends on the role of the facilitator and their attributes and skills).

Successful implementation will occur 'when evidence is scientifically robust and matches professional consensus and patients' preferences ... the context receptive to change with sympathetic cultures, strong leadership, and appropriate monitoring and feedback systems ... and, when there is appropriate facilitation of change with input from skilled external and internal facilitators.' (pp. 112–13).

This framework may be used to diagnose the receptiveness of each context to change and thereby tailor any facilitation to meet the needs of that specific context.

OTTAWA MODEL OF RESEARCH USE (OMRU) (LOGAN AND GRAHAM, 2010)

This model specifically focuses on getting valid research findings implemented.

There are six key structural elements:
- the research-informed innovation
- the potential adopters
- the practice environment
- implementation interventions for transferring the research findings into practice
- the adoption of the innovation
- the outcomes – health-related and others.

In addition there are three process elements (AME) that need to be considered – **A**ssessment of barriers and supports (which are associated with structural elements 1–3 above), **M**onitoring how the research-informed innovation is implemented, and **E**valuation of the impact of the innovation (monitoring and evaluation being linked closely to structural elements 4–6).

This model can be applied to evidence-based practice projects and also quality improvement projects.

KNOWLEDGE-TO-ACTION (KTA) FRAMEWORK (GRAHAM AND TETROE, 2010)

This framework is conceptually robust, being derived from an analysis of 31 planned action/change theories in health and social sciences, education and management.

The framework emphasises the importance of social interaction and of tailoring evidence to meet contextual and cultural needs.

The framework comprises a number of phases:
- identify problem/ select knowledge
- adapt knowledge to the local context
- assess barriers to knowledge use
- implement tailored intervention
- monitor knowledge use
- evaluate outcomes (those associated with both the process of change and the outcomes in relation to healthcare)
- sustain knowledge use.

JOANNA BRIGGS INSTITUTE (JBI) FRAMEWORK FOR IMPLEMENTING EVIDENCE (PEARSON, 2010)

This framework is particularly focused on the use of research evidence.

At its core, there are four key components:
- healthcare evidence generation
- evidence synthesis
- evidence/knowledge transfer
- evidence utilisation.

Our primary concern is the use of evidence – this part of the framework focuses on practice change, embedding evidence through system/ organisation-wide change and evaluating its impact.

The framework emphasises that the process of evidence utilisation is influenced by:
- resources
- education/expertise
- patient preference
- the availability of research
- staffing levels, skill mix
- policies.

In addition, many practitioners and researchers are now encouraging the use of more participative research designs (e.g. action research, practitioner research or engaged scholarship) (see the Activity). These forge early partnerships between researchers and practitioners that may lead to a closer match between the research needs of practitioners and the research generated for use, thereby helping research to move more quickly and effectively into practice. In addition to these sorts of partnership, nurses should be encouraged to develop their own research skills and knowledge.

FINDING MORE OUT ABOUT RESEARCH AND CHANGE MANAGEMENT

Read the following to find more out about these ideas.

Action research

Go to any research textbook and look up action research. If you don't already have a research book, a good place to start is: Depoy E, Gitlin L (2010) *Introduction to Research: Understanding and applying multiple strategies*, 4th edn. St Louis: CV Mosby.

Practitioner research

Read the chapter by Brendan McCormack on practitioner research in Hardy S, Titchen A, McCormack B, Manley K (2009) *Revealing Nursing Expertise through Practitioner Inquiry*. Oxford: Wiley-Blackwell.

Engaged scholarship

Read this paper by Brendan McCormack (2011): Engaged scholarship and research impact: integrating the doing and using of research in practice. *Journal of Research in Nursing* 16(2): 111–27.

Techniques to help change practice

Go to the National Institute for Health Research Service Delivery and Organisation programme website – http://www.sdo.nihr.ac.uk – and look at:

- the publications dropdown menu under 'News, publications & events'; then go to 'Managing change in the NHS'. There you will find a series of useful and easy to read reports;
- the research publications available around change. You will find these when you type 'change management' into the search facility.

Closely linked to research utilisation is the development of oneself and others in order to find, use and evaluate the best possible evidence for the delivery of high-quality care. The next section focuses on this type of development.

The ongoing development of oneself and others

There are many ways, some more familiar to you than others, through which you will develop yourself and other people as you practise nursing. Although we tend to think about these and describe them in what often seem to be fairly discrete, concrete chunks, for example preceptorship, mentoring, continuing professional development (CPD), clinical supervision (CS) and practice development, most learning about ourselves and our practice takes place informally as we talk together about care and our experiences in what are known as communities of practice (CoPs; le May, 2009b; Wenger, 1998). This section highlights the essentials of these activities, points out any relevant guidance from professional and statutory bodies and gives you some ideas for further reading. The final subsection sets you a challenge – to be as creative as you can in order to develop yourself and other people – and offers you some ideas to stimulate your creativity.

PRECEPTORSHIP

It has been known for nearly 40 years that some people will find moving from being a student to being a registered nurse extremely challenging (Kramer, 1974). In order to minimise the reality shock associated with this time of transition, a period of what has become known as preceptorship is recommended by, among others, the NMC, the Department of Health (DH) and the RCN.

Preceptorship is 'a period of structured transition for newly registered practitioners during which [time] he or she will be supported by a preceptor, to develop their confidence as an autonomous professional, refine skills, values and behaviours and to continue on their journey to life-long learning' (Department of Health, 2010a, p. 11). The NMC definition of preceptorship (see the Professional Guidelines box) is more specific to nursing.

PROFESSIONAL GUIDELINES

NURSING AND MIDWIFERY COUNCIL (NMC) INFORMATION ABOUT PRECEPTORSHIP (2006)

The NMC circular (21/2006) detailing preceptorship requirements defines preceptorship as being:

about providing support and guidance enabling 'new registrants' to make the transition from student to accountable practitioner to:

- *practise in accordance with the NMC code of professional conduct: standards for conduct, performance and ethics;*
- *develop confidence in their competence as a nurse, midwife or specialist community public health nurse;*

To facilitate this the 'new registrant' should have:

- *learning time protected in their first year of qualified practice; and*
- *have access to a preceptor with whom regular meetings are held.*

(http://www.nmc-uk.org/Documents/Circulars/2006circulars/NMC%20circular%2021_2006.pdf)

In 2010, the DH updated its Good Practice Guidance on preceptorship, emphasising the importance of ensuring the smoothest possible transition from student to qualified nurse (Department of Health, 2010a). The quality of this transition impacts not only on each individual nurse's job satisfaction and ability to provide safe and effective care, but also on the stability of the nursing workforce. This latter point is important to employers as a smooth transition at this point in a nurse's career is likely to mean that fewer nurses will leave the profession or remain within it feeling unsupported and disillusioned.

During your period of preceptorship (usually around 4 months) you will work with a preceptor (a nurse who has been qualified for at least a year) who will enable you to (Department of Health, 2010a):

- further develop your confidence;
- socialise you into your working environment;
- feel valued within your working environment;
- further develop your understanding of the commitment to working within professional and regulatory body requirements;
- recognise your responsibility for maintaining up-to-date knowledge.

The Professional Guidelines box details the characteristics of a successful preceptor as identified by the DoH (2010a).

PROFESSIONAL GUIDELINES

THE CHARACTERISTICS OF AN EFFECTIVE PRECEPTOR
Effective preceptors should be able to

- give constructive feedback;
- set goals and assess competency;
- facilitate problem-solving;
- use active listening skills;
- understand, demonstrate and evidence reflective-practice ability in the working environment;
- demonstrate good time-management and leadership skills;
- prioritise care;
- demonstrate appropriate clinical decision-making and evidence-based practice;
- recognise their own limitations and those of others;
- know what resources are available and how to refer a newly registered practitioner appropriately if additional support is required, for example pastoral support or occupational health services;
- be an effective and inspirational role model and demonstrate professional values, attitudes and behaviours;
- demonstrate a clear understanding of the regulatory impact of the care that they deliver and have the ability to pass on this knowledge;
- provide a high standard of practice at all times.

(Department of Health, 2010a, p. 17)

Your period of preceptorship is likely to include your being involved in many different types of learning, ranging from self-directed study (have a look at this Scottish online development programme for newly qualified nurses: http://www.flyingstart.scot.nhs.uk) to group learning and individual coaching and support.

The NMC is campaigning to make a period of preceptorship mandatory as part of its revalidation project (a project designed to determine, by 2014, how nurses and midwives demonstrate that their skills and knowledge are up to date and relevant to their area of practice). This campaign is based on the firm belief that if nurses are well supported during this time of transition, they will be more likely to settle effectively into their new role as a registered nurse; they may also gain valuable experiences and knowledge for their future development as a mentor or preceptor to others.

MENTORSHIP

Having a mentor, a guiding teacher, is something that you are familiar with – you have worked alongside one throughout your practice placements so it should be easy for you to identify the main characteristics of successful mentoring. What you will not be so familiar with is being one yourself. This section is designed to help you consider what being a mentor might entail in preparation for your post-registration responsibilities in relation to helping students learn in practice.

ACTIVITY

WHAT MAKES A GOOD MENTOR?

Reflect on your experiences of being mentored in your practice placements and jot down the answers to the following questions:

- What do you think are the most important characteristics of a good mentor?
- What did mentors do to enable you to learn successfully?
- How could the mentors that you have worked with have made your learning more successful?

Consider these features as you read this section of the text.

Although the NMC states that all students have to work with a mentor during their practical placements, you will find that many people, regardless of their job, have informal mentors who guide and advise them throughout their careers – the guiding teacher that we referred to at the start of this section. You may also already have discovered that you have a talent for guiding other people in their learning, be they your peers and more junior students or others in your everyday life, and it is these skills that you will go on to develop both formally as an NMC mentor and more informally as people begin to trust you and respect your competence. Mentoring is all about helping people to learn to do things and supporting them in their experience of learning.

The responsibilities of an NMC mentor relate very specifically to the determination of every mentee's competence and ability to practise safely; as a qualified nurse, you will be required to mentor students and assess their competence in practice. At the time of writing, the NMC's (2008a) standards provide details of how to support learning and assessment in practice, including how mentorship should be carried out as well as the competencies that a mentor must achieve (see the Professional Guidelines boxes).

PROFESSIONAL GUIDELINES

RESPONSIBILITIES OF AN NMC MENTOR

Mentors are responsible and accountable for:

- Organising and co-ordinating student learning activities in practice.
- Supervising students in learning situations and providing them with constructive feedback on their achievements.
- Setting and monitoring achievement of realistic learning objectives.
- Assessing total performance – including skills, attitudes and behaviours.
- Providing evidence as required by programme providers of student achievement or lack of achievement.
- Liaising with others (e.g. mentors, sign-off mentors, practice facilitators, practice teachers, personal tutors, programme leaders) to provide feedback, identify any concerns about the student's performance and agree action as appropriate.
- Providing evidence for, or acting as, sign-off mentors with regard to making decisions about achievement of proficiency at the end of a programme.

(Nursing and Midwifery Council, 2008a, p.21)

PROFESSIONAL GUIDELINES

COMPETENCE AND OUTCOMES FOR A MENTOR

Establishing effective working relationships

- Demonstrate an understanding of factors that influence how students integrate into practice settings.
- Provide ongoing and constructive support to facilitate transition from one learning environment to another.
- Have effective professional and interprofessional working relationships to support learning for entry to the register.

Facilitation of learning

- Use knowledge of the student's stage of learning to select appropriate learning opportunities to meet individual needs.
- Facilitate the selection of appropriate learning strategies to integrate learning from practice and academic experiences.
- Support students in critically reflecting upon their learning experiences in order to enhance future learning.

Assessment and accountability

- Foster professional growth, personal development and accountability through support of students in practice.
- Demonstrate a breadth of understanding of assessment strategies and the ability to contribute to the total assessment process as part of the teaching team.
- Provide constructive feedback to students and assist them in identifying future learning needs and actions. Manage failing students so that they may enhance their performance and capabilities for safe and effective practice or be able to understand their failure and the implications of this for their future.
- Be accountable for confirming that students have met, or not met, the NMC competencies in practice. As a sign-off mentor confirm that students have met, or not met, the NMC standards of proficiency in practice and are capable of safe and effective practice.

Evaluation of learning

- Contribute to evaluation of student learning and assessment experiences – proposing aspects for change resulting from such evaluation.
- Participate in self and peer evaluation to facilitate personal development, and contribute to the development of others.

Creating an environment for learning

- Support students to identify both learning needs and experiences that are appropriate to their level of learning.
- Use a range of learning experiences, involving patients, clients, carers and the professional team, to meet defined learning needs.
- Identify aspects of the learning environment which could be enhanced – negotiating with others to make appropriate changes.
- Act as a resource to facilitate personal and professional development of others.

Context of practice

- Contribute to the development of an environment in which effective practice is fostered, implemented, evaluated and disseminated.
- Set and maintain professional boundaries that are sufficiently flexible for providing interprofessional care.
- Initiate and respond to practice developments to ensure safe and effective care is achieved and an effective learning environment is maintained.

Evidence-based practice

- Identify and apply research and evidence-based practice to their area of practice.
- Contribute to strategies to increase or review the evidence base used to support practice.
- Support students in applying an evidence base to their own practice.

Leadership

- **Plan a series of learning experiences that will meet students' defined learning needs.**
- **Be an advocate for students to support them accessing learning opportunities that meet their individual needs – involving a range of other professionals, patients, clients and carers.**
- **Prioritise work to accommodate support of students within their practice roles.**
- **Provide feedback about the effectiveness of learning and assessment in practice.**

(Nursing and Midwifery Council, 2008a, p. 20–1)

In order to achieve these, you will first have to undertake and pass a post-registration course on mentoring. This course, coupled with your experience, will enable you to help students understand practice better, and link theory, research and practice together more easily. To enable you to do this, you will need to have a wide collection of complementary skills, which will include:

- being able to communicate clearly the relationships between theory, research and practice that underpin the student's (your mentee's) learning;
- teaching people, using a variety of techniques, either as you work alongside your mentee or more formally with groups of students on your ward/unit;
- helping your mentee to gain practice skills and knowledge;
- coaching and supporting in order to build your mentee's confidence and competence;
- assessing practice and your mentee's development;
- encouraging your mentee to reflect on their practice and identify aspects of it that have gone well or not gone so well, as well as to determine why;
- being able to provide constructive yet critical feedback;
- being able to liaise with others in the education team and report accurately on your mentee's progress;
- learning with your mentee (often nurses say that they most enjoy mentoring students because they learn from and with them);
- acting as a role model or – to take a concept from the earlier section on leadership – mentoring often requires you to 'model the way' (Kouzes and Posner, 2002) and show your mentee (and of course others whom you work with) how to do things through their observing your own behaviour and attitudes.

Being a mentor is an important aspect of your own and others' development. Mentoring not only offers you opportunities to continuously improve your own practice by seeking out and using the latest research and actively discussing your practice with other people, but also offers some degree of personal satisfaction as you engage in the development of other people.

Go and read The *Nurse Mentor's Handbook: Supporting students in clinical practice*, by D. Walsh (2010)
Maidenhead: Open University Press.
This book will provide you with a wealth of valuable information about teaching and learning theories,
teaching and assessing in practice and how to support students who are not doing well or failing.
There are useful hints on how to prepare and present teaching sessions, including tips on PowerPoint
presentations. The book also provides useful information on how to make the best of placements that
you find challenging, and has a chapter on 'Helping a student survive a placement'.

ACTIVITY

CONTINUING PROFESSIONAL DEVELOPMENT

CPD is something that every healthcare professional is responsible for doing. Making sure that you continually develop your knowledge and skills through CPD is essential to the maintenance of a safe and appropriately skilled health and social care workforce that can deliver the best possible care to people.

The NMC (2010) lays down particular requirements for CPD in order for nurses to maintain their registration. These requirements must be met every time you renew your registration. There are many ways to maintain your professional development, ranging from undertaking courses to presenting information at conferences about work that you are doing in practice or through research to belonging to various specialist interest groups or action learning sets. Although this type of CPD is often associated with developing your clinical knowledge and skills, it is important that you also pay attention to developing alternative skills that will, in turn, enhance the care that you provide, for example becoming more assertive, developing the ability to delegate to others and developing the ability to say no when you feel overburdened. Paying attention to these sorts of developmental need is critical to creating an environment within which your patients, your colleagues and yourself will all flourish. To take account of the breadth of CPD activities, you might see CPD described as continuing personal and professional development (CPPD).

Very closely linked to CPD, in my mind, is CS (clinical supervision). CS offers all nurses the opportunity to learn through reflecting on their experience of day-to-day practice with an experienced colleague; this learning, once acted upon, has the potential to enhance the quality of subsequent practice. Lyth (2000), following a concept analysis of clinical supervision, offered the following definition.

> Clinical supervision is a support mechanism for practising professionals within which they can share clinical, organizational, developmental and emotional experiences with another professional in a secure, confidential environment in order to enhance knowledge and skills. This process will lead to an increased awareness of other concepts including accountability and reflective practice. (p. 729)

The NMC (2008b) has set out a set of principles to underpin clinical supervision, which are outlined in the Professional Guidelines box. Clinical supervision is intricately linked not only to one's own continuous development, but also to the ongoing development of practice. The next section gives you some ideas about changing practice.

PRINCIPLES UNDERPINNING CLINICAL SUPERVISION

- Clinical supervision supports practice, enabling registered nurses to maintain and improve standards of care
- Clinical supervision is a practice-focused professional relationship, involving a practitioner reflecting on practice guided by a skilled supervisor
- Registered nurses and managers should develop the process of clinical supervision according to local circumstances. Ground rules should be agreed so that the supervisor and the registered nurse approach clinical supervision openly, confidently and are aware of what is involved
- Every registered nurse should have access to clinical supervision and each supervisor should supervise a realistic number of practitioners
- Preparation for supervisors should be flexible and sensitive to local circumstances. The principles and relevance of clinical supervision should be included in pre-registration and post-registration education programmes
- Evaluation of clinical supervision is needed to assess how it influences care and practice standards. Evaluation systems should be determined locally.

(Nursing and Midwifery Council, 2008b)

PRACTICE DEVELOPMENT

Practice development is about supporting positive change within practice in order to improve patient care and the working environment within which care is given; this process essentially involves learning, changing and evaluating. I am including practice development in this section because, for me, it not only builds on many of the aspects of personal development and the development of others that have just been discussed, but also unites the four central themes of Chapters 3 and 4 within the reality of practice. Practice development offers individuals, teams and organisations opportunities to do things differently and creatively.

Practice development is defined as:

> a continuous process of improvement towards increased effectiveness in patient-centred care. This is brought about by helping healthcare teams to develop their knowledge and skills and to transform the culture and context of care. It is enabled and supported by facilitators committed to systematic rigorous continuous processes of emancipatory change that reflect the perspectives of service users and service providers. (Garbett and McCormack, 2002; quoted in McCormack, 2009, p. 45)

Practice development is not a new idea. It has been with us for a long time but only started to gain prominence in nursing during the 1980s with the creation of nursing development units and the changing political and professional emphasis favouring nurse-led care. Of course, you do not need either a designated 'development' unit to develop practice or a focus on care led by nurses – what you do need, though, is support from colleagues, managers and other stakeholders, as well as fearless enthusiasm. This latter quality is evident in the career sketch that Brendan McCormack – a well-known and respected proponent of practice development – wrote (shown here).

BRENDAN McCORMACK'S CAREER

I kind of 'fell into' nursing as my school education programme was very much geared towards me being an engineer (something I knew I never wanted to be) and began my nursing life as a psychiatric nurse in Ireland. However I was totally unprepared for the experience and the life-change it would mean for me. I was quite shocked at the level of institutionalised abuse that existed and by the lack of humanity. But it is these memories that have driven most of the things I have since done in nursing and still feel passionate about, i.e. that it is easy to slip into institutionalised, routinised and thoughtless ways of practising if the culture is not one that is vigilant and unrelenting about quality and enables real engagement in the ongoing transformation of that culture.

Over the years, the whole idea of facilitating practice knowledge and working with adult learning approaches to transforming lives has really excited me, and my work in practice development and practitioner research has enabled me to realise that excitement. My career has been unusual and I have not followed what I see as a typical academic career – indeed I struggle with the 'academic' label as my passion is 'practice' and have spent most of my career in joint-appointments as I firmly believe that we need to be alongside practitioners and decision-makers if we are going to have real and sustained impact. I have been influenced by the work of Paulo Freire, Karl Rogers, John Heron and a host of creative scholars who have enabled me to be eclectic in how I approach my work.

I have always been 'on the edge' methodologically as I refuse to exist in an epistemological box! Because of that position, I have been able to experiment with a variety of methodologies that integrate learning, development and research. The use of creative arts as an integral part of that experimentation has become central to how I work – it is not about being an artist, but instead is a way of finding non-cognitive processes of engagement, learning and analysing thorny questions. I have worked with my colleague Professor Angie Titchen in the development of a new theoretical and methodological framework called 'Critical Creativity' – an approach that integrates the 'critical' with the 'creative'. I work with a range of research and practice development projects that utilise this methodology and with a number of doctoral students who are the 'new experimenters' with non-formulaic research! I love the look on my colleagues' faces when I talk about 'dancing my data!'

Nursing needs left-of-centre thinkers and experimenters. We live in a world that is dominated by protocols, guidelines, performance-measures, targets and rules, all of which serve to make us all the same and eliminate risky practice – without taking risk we never change and we will always get more of the same. As my hero Oscar Wilde said, 'We are all in the gutter, but some of us are looking at the stars.'

(Professor Brendan McCormack, DPhil (Oxon), BSc (Hons), PGCEA, RNT, RMN, RGN; Director, Institute of Nursing Research and Head of the Person-centred Practice Research Centre, University of Ulster, Northern Ireland; Adjunct Professor of Nursing, University of Technology, Sydney; Adjunct Professor of Nursing, Faculty of Medicine, Nursing and Health Care, Monash University, Melbourne; Visiting Professor, School of Medicine and Dentistry, University of Aberdeen; Professor II, Buskerud University College, Drammen, Norway)

McCormack et al.'s (2006) review of the available knowledge on practice development draws out the key characteristics and components of practice development projects (Box 4.7). This is a comprehensive review, and some of you might like to read it all at http://www.nhshealthquality.org/nhsqis/files/Final%20report.pdf. This review makes clear the potential of practice development to really make a difference to the quality of care that people receive, and to the quality of the working environments within which nurses and other health and social care professionals provide care – in other words to change workplace cultures in their entirety. This is taken further in a later publication (Manley et al., 2009), which explores more widely the knowledge base of practice development and its critical application to practice.

BOX 4.7 KEY CHARACTERISTICS/COMPONENTS OF PRACTICE DEVELOPMENT PROJECTS

Practice development projects should be able to demonstrate evidence of using all the following methods:

- Agreed ethical processes
- Stakeholder analysis and agreed ways of engaging stakeholders
- Person-centredness
- Values clarification
- Developing a shared vision
- Workplace culture analysis
- Collaboration and participation
- Developing shared ownership
- Reflective learning
- Methods to facilitate critical reflection (e.g. action learning)
- High challenge and high support
- Feedback
- Knowledge use
- Process and outcome evaluation
- Facilitation of transitions
- Giving space for ideas to flourish
- Dissemination of learning

McCormack et al., 2006, p.11

Everyone can be involved in developing practice no matter how large or small the change that is planned. And although the theoretical side of it might seem overwhelming, when you read around it the benefits for patients can be enormous. Some of these benefits (and a realisation that there is still progress to be made) are captured in a paper by McCormack in the *Journal of Research in Nursing* (2011, p. 120). Here he discusses a practice development programme based on the idea of engaged scholarship. The programme, still ongoing, focuses on the creation of a person-centred culture in the care of older people. Here is an extract from the paper that shows their progress and some areas still to be addressed:

For residents and families, the data demonstrated significant changes in care practices that resulted in an impact on four key areas of care experiences for older people and their families, with each of them showing qualitatively a change in the practice culture:

- Hope and Hopelessness: … the data shows a shift towards increased hopefulness in the way that residents are cared for, including the range of activities available for residents, their involvement in decision-making and the quality of engagements between staff and residents. However, hopelessness among residents continues to be an issue and one that needs further work.
- Choice: The data demonstrated that residents were provided with a greater range and number of choices. Specific activities (such as resident and family groups) have been initiated and established in the majority of settings as methods of enabling more choice for residents.
- Belonging and Connectedness: There was evidence of staff 'knowing the person' in a more meaningful way in this data set compared with Year 1 data. A range of activities have been initiated to enable greater knowing of residents as persons with 'histories' and these can be seen to have had an impact on the quality and quantity of meaningful engagement with residents. A lot of attention has been paid to improving the environment in many of the participating sites and this has been viewed positively.
- Meaningful relationships: The attention paid to such issues (which are overt demonstrations of being more person-centred) as language, team-work, reducing ritual and routine, facilitating more choice, intentionality and the development of meaningful relationships has had a positive impact on resident experience.

This extract clearly illustrates how practice development can make a difference to people – the challenge for everyone is how to sustain that change once it has been made.

ACTIVITY

FINDING OUT ABOUT THE REALITIES OF PRACTICE DEVELOPMENT

Ask around your local hospital or community nursing team and find out if you have a practice development facilitator or coordinator working there. If there is one, arrange to talk to them and find out about what they do. Ask them about the projects they are involved in, and see if they will let you shadow them for a short period of time to find out more. If you can't find a specific person, ask around and find out where your colleagues or your mentor think practice development is occurring and go and visit that unit or team.

See how the projects compare with the characteristics of practice development projects that McCormack et al. noted (see Box 4.8).

COMMUNITIES OF PRACTICE

As already mentioned, much of our learning and exchange of ideas happens in groups with other people. Over the last decade or so, these groups have been called CoPs (Wenger, 1998). CoPs are:

> groups of people who share a concern, a set of problems, or a passion about a topic, and who deepen their understanding and knowledge of this area by interacting on an ongoing basis. ... These people don't necessarily work together on a day-to-day basis, but they get together because they find value in their interactions. As they spend time together, they typically share information, insight, and advice. They solve problems. They help each other. They discuss their situation, their aspirations, their needs. They think about common issues. They explore ideas and act as sounding boards to each other. They may create tools, standards, generic designs, manuals, and other documents; or they may just keep what they know as a tacit understanding they share. ... Over time, they develop a unique perspective on their topic as well as a body of common knowledge, practices, and approaches. They also develop personal relationships and established ways of interacting. They may even develop a common sense of identity. They become a community of practice. (Wenger et al., 2002, pp. 4–5)

CoPs are ideal ways to get people together in order to share knowledge, reflect on experiences, learn from each other and discuss the best ways to implement knowledge or shape old knowledge for new practices in order to suit the needs and context of their area of practice or particular patients.

Additionally, CoPs have the potential to impact positively on the 'standard of care delivered to patients/clients; working environments and job satisfaction of the participants in the community; speed with which problems are solved; speed with which knowledge and innovation moves into practice; creation of a unified team which may be uni- or multi-professional; ownership and sustainability of changes to practice' (le May, 2009b, p. 4). An extra advantage is that they can function either as real face-to-face communities or virtually via interactive learning environments or electronic discussion groups. Ask around and see if you can find some CoPs in the organisation that you work in – find out what they do and think about whether or not you could create one around an area that you are interested in, or alternatively whether you could join one that is already established.

DEVELOPING ENTREPRENEURIAL SKILLS

The penultimate section of this chapter focuses on something that is becoming increasingly important to the development of nursing and patient care – the development of entrepreneurial skills. First linked explicitly to nursing in the debates surrounding the modernising of nursing careers that started in 2006 (Department of Health, 2006) nurses were encouraged to become more entrepreneurial in their work within the NHS. This development stemmed from a change in the law enabling nurses to become partners in general practices and run nurse-led primary care services. Since then, the new coalition government has re-emphasised its intention to promote social enterprise; indeed, its 'ambition is to create the largest and most vibrant social enterprise sector in the world' (Department of Health, 2010b, p. 5), reigniting the need for the development of entrepreneurial skills in all healthcare professionals.

Some of you might be wondering how entrepreneurship and nursing actually go together. Surely, you are thinking, being an entrepreneur is about creating new businesses? Well to a certain extent you are right, and although nurses are quite able and are indeed being encouraged to do this through the promotion of social enterprises, the majority of you will focus on another side of entrepreneurship – being innovative. Those of you who think your career path might lie with the combination of business development and innovation will be inspired by reading Sarah Chilver's description of her career here, and maybe by visiting her company's website at http://www.chilversmccrea.co.uk.

SARAH CHILVERS

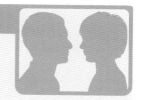

Sarah Chilvers, at the age of 19, was not sure which direction to turn. A levels under her belt and a passionate interest in health, wellbeing and all things medical, she decided to go into an 'academic type of nursing' – one of the first degrees in Nursing in the UK. This done and several babies later (she now has eight children), Sarah set off into the world of community nursing/health visiting, utterly frustrated with the NHS and feeling there ought to be ways of doing things more effectively, differently and better for patients. None of this was a criticism of her fellow clinicians (perhaps of the system), it was more an energy and enthusiasm to improve the way that things were done. Nor did she ever assume that the models she developed would be an answer for the whole of the NHS, so her approach has always been to problem solve where there were problems and always seek learning and improvement. All of this passion took Sarah on a pathway to piloting programmes of care for people who would traditionally be cared for in hospital, out into their homes, it took her to initiating new and innovative ways of providing cancer services, it brought her into involving patients and providing better information for people using services, and most notably recently she has set up (in 2001) and now merged the company ChilversMcCrea Ltd (CML) with a trade partner (2010). Many of these ventures won Sarah national awards including the IPPR Guardian award for public involvement and the Entrepreneur of the Year award from Laing and Buisson. CML was the first company of its kind to run GP practices using a commercial and corporate approach. Whilst it actually didn't differ from other GP practice models the difference came through the scale of the project. The business rose to 40 practices and a turnover of over £15 million. Sarah is now working with the same pioneering GP and business partner, Rory McCrea, to develop community services that will be of interest and relevance to the GP consortia as they take responsibility for commissioning a new suite of NHS services more cost effectively than ever before. 'We believe our model provides excellent care to people more cost effectively than hospital options ... the key to success with any venture such as this is always team work!!!'

Watch this space ... Sarah Chilvers is now Director of ChilversMcCrea Healthcare and has a doctorate from Middlesex University that involved researching innovative models of provision in primary care, as well as an MBA from the Open University. Her first degree was a BSc (Hons) in Nursing from Chelsea College (now King's College), London University, and she still actively maintains her registration on both the first and second levels of the NMC Register.

For the vast majority of you, becoming more entrepreneurial will be largely about using the skills of an entrepreneur in your day-to-day practice in order to be more innovative. The UK Centre for Bioscience at the University of Leeds has identified a wide range of skills needed by entrepreneurs (Box 4.8) and also by people who want to be entrepreneurial within an existing organisation (an 'intrapreneur'). Look at their website http://www.bioscience.heacademy.ac.uk/resources/entrepreneurship/skills.aspx for more information, and read the paper by Hewison and Badger (2006) on nurse intrapreneurs in the NHS. Using these skills will make you think differently, and thinking differently will enable you to have a greater degree of freedom to take the risks that Brendan McCormack suggests we are sometimes reluctant to take.

BOX 4.8 ENTREPRENEURIAL SKILLS

Entrepreneurial skills include:

- Management skills – the ability to manage time and people (both yourself and others) successfully
- Communication skills and the ability to sell ideas and persuade others
- The ability to work both as part of a team and independently
- Being able to plan, coordinate and organise effectively
- Financial literacy
- Being able to research effectively, e.g. available markets, suppliers, customers and the competition
- Self-motivation and discipline
- Being adaptable
- Innovative thinking and being creative
- The ability to multitask
- Being able to take responsibility and make decisions
- The ability to work under pressure
- Perseverance
- Competitiveness
- Willingness to take risks
- Having the ability to network and make contacts

UK Centre for Bioscience; http://www.bioscience.heacademy.ac.uk/resources/entrepreneurship/skills.aspx

Thinking differently

The whole point of this book is to inspire you to see the range of opportunities that a nursing career offers and to give you ideas about how you might expertly practise nursing. Thinking differently about your practice might require you to be more creative than you think you can be and sometimes take measured risks, not only in the ways by which you give high-quality, evidence-based, expert care, but also in the opportunities you select in order to develop yourself and other people as your career progresses.

Creativity can take many forms in nursing – you have already come across some of them in this chapter, and as you read on into the second part of this book, you will come across others. In many instances, being creative may simply be bringing together the many sources of knowledge and skills that you have in a new way in order to provide the best care to each person whom you are nursing. This level of creativity will require you to use what are termed clinical mindlines (Gabbay and le May, 2011):

> internalized, collectively reinforced and often tacit guidelines that are informed by clinicians' training, by their own and each others' experience, by their interactions with their role sets, by their reading, by the way they have learnt to handle [their] conflicting demands, by their understanding of local circumstances and systems, and by a host of other sources … Clinicians build up mindlines as a bank of personalized, flexible syntheses of all the different types of theoretical and experiential knowledge that they need to be able to call upon instantaneously. (p. 43–4)

In other instances, being creative may require you to take a leap into uncertainty in order to create and lead innovative, person-centred, high-quality care for patients and service users that uses the most up-to-date and relevant research available; doing this successfully is the challenge that all nurses face. You will see in the second half of this book how some nurses have taken up this challenge, and we hope that their stories will inspire you to be creative and to develop your own brand of expert practice as your careers progress.

References

Adair J (2010) *Not Bosses but Leaders*, 3rd edn. London: Kogan Page.

Binney G, Wilke G, Williams C (2005) *Living Leadership: A practical guide for ordinary heroes*. Harlow: Prentice-Hall

Cox Y, le May A (2007) Leadership for practice. In: *Principles of Professional Studies in Nursing*, Brown J, Libberton P (eds). Basingstoke: Palgrave Macmillan, pp. 155–71.

Cullum N, Cilisha D, Maynes B, Marks S (2008) *Evidence-based Nursing: An introduction*. Oxford: Blackwell.

Daft R (1999) *Leadership Theory and Practice*. Fort Worth, TX: Harcourt Brace.

Department of Health (2006) *Modernising Nursing Careers – Setting the Direction*. London: DH.

Department of Health (2010a) *Preceptorship Framework for Newly Registered Nurses, Midwives and Allied Health Professionals*. London: DH.

Department of Health (2010b) *Equity and Excellence: Liberating the NHS*. London: DH.

Gabbay J, le May A (2011) *Practice Based Evidence for Healthcare: Clinical mindlines*. London: Routledge.

Garbett R, McCormack B (2002) A concept analysis of practice development. *NT Research* 7(2): 87–100.

Graham I, Tetroe J (2010) The knowledge to action framework. In: *Models and Frameworks for Implementing Evidence-Based Practice: Linking evidence to action*, Rycroft-Malone J, Bucknall T (eds). Oxford: Wiley-Blackwell, pp. 207–22.

Handy C (1993) *Understanding Organizations*. Harmondsworth: Penguin.

Hersey P, Blanchard K (1977) *Management of Organizational Behavior – Utilizing Human Resources*. Englewood Cliffs, NJ: Prentice Hall.

Hewison A, Badger F (2006) Taking the initiative: nurse intrapreneurs in the NHS. *Nursing Management* 13(3): 14–19.

Kouzes J, Posner B (2002) *The Leadership Challenge*. San Francisco: Jossey-Bass.

Kramer M (1974) *Reality Shock: Why nurses leave nursing*. St Louis: CV Mosby.

le May A (1999) *Evidence Based Practice*. Nursing Times Clinical Monograph No. 1. London: EMAP.

le May A (2009a) Introducing communities of practice designed to develop older people's services. In: *Communities of Practice in Health and Social Care*, pp. 3–16. Oxford: Blackwell

le May A (2009b) Generating patient capital: the contribution of story telling in communities of practice designed to develop older people's services. In: *Communities of Practice in Health and Social Care*. Oxford: Blackwell, pp. 95–106.

le May A, Mulhall A, Alexander C (1998) Bridging the research-practice gap: exploring the research cultures of practitioners and managers. *Journal of Advanced Nursing* 28(2): 428–37.

Logan J, Graham I (2010) The Ottawa model of research use. In: *Models and Frameworks for Implementing Evidence-Based Practice: Linking evidence to action*, Rycroft-Malone J, Bucknall T (eds). Oxford: Wiley-Blackwell, pp. 83–136.

London Regional Office (2000) *Embodying Leadership*. London: Department of Health.

Lyth G (2000) Clinical supervision: a concept analysis. *Journal of Advanced Nursing* 31(3): 722–9.

McCormack B (2009) Practitioner research. In: *Revealing Nursing Expertise Through Practitioner Inquiry*, Hardy S, Titchen A, McCormack B, Manley K (eds). Oxford: Wiley-Blackwell, pp. 31–54.

McCormack B (2011) Engaged scholarship and research impact: integrating the doing and using of research in practice. *Journal of Research in Nursing* 16(2): 111–27.

McCormack B, Dewar B, Wright J, Garbett R, Harvey G, Ballantine K (2006) *A Realist Synthesis of Evidence Relating to Practice Development: Final Report to NHS Education For Scotland and NHS Quality Improvement Scotland*. Retrieved from: http://www.nhshealthquality.org/nhsqis/files/Final%20report.pdf (accessed 2 January 2011).

McNichol E, Hamer S (2006) *Leadership and Management: A 3-dimensional approach*. Cheltenham: Nelson Thornes.

Manley K, Titchen A, Hardy S (2009) From artistry in practice to expertise in developing person-centred systems: a clinical career framework. In: *Revealing Nursing Expertise Through Practitioner Inquiry*, Hardy S, Titchen A, McCormack B, Manley K (eds). Oxford: Wiley-Blackwell, pp. 3–30.

Mullins L (1999) *Management and Organisational Behaviour*. Harlow: Prentice-Hall.

NHS Leadership Centre (2002) *The NHS Leadership Qualities Framework*. London: Department of Health.

Nursing and Midwifery Council (2006) *Preceptorship Guidelines*. Circular 21/2006. Retrieved from: http://www.nmc-uk.org/Documents/Circulars/2006circulars/NMC%20circular%2021_2006.pdf (accessed 2 January 2011).

Nursing and Midwifery Council (2008a) Standards to Support Learning and Assessment in Practice NMC Standards for Mentors, Practice Teachers and Teachers. Retrieved from: http://wwwm.coventry.ac.uk/HealthcareMentors/Documents/NMC2008.pdf (accessed 2 January 2011).

Nursing and Midwifery Council (2008b) *Clinical supervision for registered nurses*. Retrieved from: http://www.nmc-uk.org/Nurses-and-midwives/Advice-by-topic/A/Advice/Clinical-supervision-for-registered-nurses/ (accessed 2 January 2011).

Nursing and Midwifery Council (2010) CPD and Practice. Retrieved from: http://www.nmc-uk.org/Employers-and-managers/Your-responsibilities/CPD-and-practice/ (accessed 2 January 2011).

Pearson A (2010) The Joanna Briggs Institute model of evidence-based health care as a framework for implementing evidence. In: *Models and Frameworks for Implementing Evidence-Based Practice: Linking evidence to action*, Rycroft-Malone J, Bucknall T (eds). Oxford: Wiley-Blackwell pp. 185–205.

Rycroft-Malone J (2010) Promoting Action on Research Implementation in Health Services (PARIHS). In: *Models and Frameworks for Implementing Evidence-Based Practice: Linking evidence to action*, Rycroft-Malone J, Bucknall T (eds). Oxford: Wiley-Blackwell, pp. 109–35.

Rycroft-Malone J, Bucknall T (eds) (2010) *Models and Frameworks for Implementing Evidence-Based Practice: Linking evidence to action*. Oxford: Wiley-Blackwell.

Rycroft-Malone J, Seers K, Titchen A, Harvey G, Kitson A, McCormack B (2004) What counts as evidence in evidence-based practice? *Journal of Advanced Nursing* 47(1): 81–90.

Wenger E (1998) *Communities of Practice: learning, meaning and identity*. New York: Cambridge University Press.

Wenger E, McDermott R, Snyder W (2002) *Cultivating Communities of Practice*. Harvard, MA: Harvard Business School.